Patient-Reported Outcomes and Experience

Tim Benson

Patient-Reported Outcomes and Experience

Measuring What We Want From PROMs and PREMs

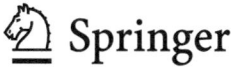

Tim Benson
R-Outcomes Ltd.
Newbury, UK

ISBN 978-3-030-97073-4   ISBN 978-3-030-97071-0 (eBook)
https://doi.org/10.1007/978-3-030-97071-0

© The Editor(s) (if applicable) and The Author(s), under exclusive license to Springer Nature Switzerland AG 2022
This work is subject to copyright. All rights are solely and exclusively licensed by the Publisher, whether the whole or part of the material is concerned, specifically the rights of translation, reprinting, reuse of illustrations, recitation, broadcasting, reproduction on microfilms or in any other physical way, and transmission or information storage and retrieval, electronic adaptation, computer software, or by similar or dissimilar methodology now known or hereafter developed.
The use of general descriptive names, registered names, trademarks, service marks, etc. in this publication does not imply, even in the absence of a specific statement, that such names are exempt from the relevant protective laws and regulations and therefore free for general use.
The publisher, the authors and the editors are safe to assume that the advice and information in this book are believed to be true and accurate at the date of publication. Neither the publisher nor the authors or the editors give a warranty, expressed or implied, with respect to the material contained herein or for any errors or omissions that may have been made. The publisher remains neutral with regard to jurisdictional claims in published maps and institutional affiliations.

This Springer imprint is published by the registered company Springer Nature Switzerland AG
The registered company address is: Gewerbestrasse 11, 6330 Cham, Switzerland

This book is dedicated to my sons Laurence, Oliver, Alex and Jamie.

Preface

The origin of this book was a paradox—why doesn't everyone use person-reported outcome and experience measures (PROMs and PREMs) if they are such a good thing? This led to detailed examination of the whole PROMs/PREMs landscape—what works, what does not and how could things that don't work be made better.

On the one hand, PROMs and PREMs can provide a key feedback loop from those who receive care to those who pay for and direct it. This feedback can benefit every level of decision-making, from patients managing their own health, doctors and nurses at the front line, managers, commissioners, policymakers and regulators.

On the other hand, routine use of PROMs and PREMs is rare outside clinical trials and a few specialty-specific examples. Where countries have sought wide implementation, success has been limited. For example, the NHS in England has required all patients having hip and knee replacement surgery to complete PROMs since 2009, but this project has not been extended.

Innovation adoption is a complex process, which can be halted by just one thing not working. Things do not have to be perfect, just good enough, but everything must work adequately. PROMs and PREMs adoption are innovations, just like the Internet and electric vehicles.

This book is aimed at many audiences.

It is aimed at the relative novice, who does not yet know what they do not know.

It is a reference and textbook, bringing together information that is known, but widely scattered across academic journals. Too often projects come to grief by failing to learn hard-won lessons from the past.

It is also aimed at those with a good deal of experience, who like to see another point of view. I have aimed to identify things that have survived the tests of time, things that may be part of the problem and a few things that could be solutions.

The focus is on routine use of short generic PROMs and PREMs within healthcare services, not on the numerous diagnosis-specific measures that have been developed for use in clinical trials. It is aimed primarily at people providing healthcare and policymakers, not researchers in academia or the pharmaceutical business, although they may find things of interest.

This book is organised in two parts—I Principles and II Measures.

Part I focuses on principles, which apply to most PROMs and PREMs. Chapter 1 describes the nature of the problem being addressed, focusing on the widely accepted need for health and care to become more patient centred. Chapter 2 is a short history of the most significant developments up to about 2010, which are the basis for most of what we see today. Chapter 3 covers terminology, with a general discussion of the terms used within this subject area. Chapters 4 and 5 cover the barriers that need to be overcome. Some barriers are people-related (people do not like to change the way they do things), while others, such as noise and bias, are inherent in all surveys. Chapter 6 covers the general issue of how best to present the results to different people using dashboards and statistics. Chapter 7 introduces interoperability and ways to share information with people who need to know. Chapter 8 covers ways to value death and morbidity, including Quality Adjusted Life Years (QALYs), the Value of a Statistical Life (VSL) and Load paradigms.

Part II describes the main types of PROMs and PREMs where I have personal knowledge and experience. The discussion is broader than usual, covering many types of measure. The first chapter in Part II (Chap. 9) is an overview of patient-reported outcome measures in the form of a structured hierarchy. Chapter 10 covers patient experience measures and gives detailed explanations of conventions used in subsequent chapters, which are not subsequently repeated. Chapters 11 and 12 cover health status and measures of personal wellbeing, respectively. Chapter 13 covers patient-centred care, including patients' capability to manage their own health and shared decision-making (SDM). This is followed by Chap. 14 on individualised measures, where the patient states and scores what matters most to them. Chapter 15 covers social determinants of health at the individual level, social contact and loneliness. Chapter 16 covers user perceptions in the evaluation of specific healthcare innovations. Chapter 17 covers the use of PROMs and PREMs by healthcare staff. Chapter 18 covers the use by proxies where a person answers on behalf of another such as someone with dementia or a small child, by unpaid caregivers or carers and by those working or living in care homes.

If you wish to use any of the measures that I have developed (such as those shown in Chaps. 9 and 17), please contact R-Outcomes Ltd. (https://r-outcomes.com) in the first instance. These products were developed without grant-funding because I saw a need for them. Ironically, being grant-free speeded up development and focused attention on meeting market needs.

Newbury, UK Tim Benson
January 2022

Acknowledgements

Many people have contributed to the content of this book over many years: in the early days at Charing Cross Hospital, Rachel Rosser, Geoff Pegrum, Paul Kind and Ken MacRae; later, at UCL, David Ingram, Timea Helter, Justin Whatling and Seref Arikan; then Angela Coulter, Steve Sizmur, Clive Bowman, Steven Foster and Liz Dymond; and more recently Andrew Liles, Paul Gray, Henry Potts, Martin Vincent, Jess Done, Joe Sladen, Helen Seers, Alex Benson and the people at DaySix Ltd. I also want to thank all the staff and patients who have collected PROMs and PREMs and provided feedback to make them better.

Contents

I Principles

1 Why PROMs and PREMs Matter? 3
   Introduction 3
      The Quality Chasm 4
      Quality Measures 4
      What Do Health Care Systems Produce? 5
      Personalised Care 6
      PROMs and PREMs 7
      Criteria 8
   Lessons 10
   Conclusions 10
   References 11

2 History 13
   Early Pioneers 13
   PROMs 15
      Before 1980 15
      1980s 17
      1990s 18
      2000s 18
   References 19

3 Terms 21
   Descriptive Framework 21
      Questionnaire 21
      Measure 22
      Comment 24
      Readability 24
      Translations 25
   Scoring Scheme 25
      Weight 26
      Scales 27

	Conclusions	28
	References	28
4	**Why PROMs Are Hard: People**	**31**
	Response Rate	31
	Case Study—GPPS	32
	Digital Exclusion	34
	Innovation Readiness	34
	Innovativeness Spectrum	35
	Decision Process	36
	Change Management	37
	Behavior Change	38
	PDSA Cycle	40
	SMART Criteria	41
	Conclusions	42
	References	42
5	**Noise and Complexity**	**43**
	Noise and Bias	43
	Types of Noise	44
	Types of Bias	44
	Reducing Noise and Bias	46
	Complexity	48
	Complexity Theory	48
	NASSS Framework	49
	Conclusions	53
	References	53
6	**Using the Results**	**55**
	Background	55
	Analysis	56
	Roles	56
	Change	57
	Dashboard	58
	Dashboards for Managers	58
	Case Study	60
	Statistical Packages	61
	Validity	61
	Construct Validation	62
	Other Types of Validity	62
	Example	62
	Publication Check-List	63
	Conclusions	65
	References	65

7	**Sharing Data**	67
	What Is Interoperability	67
	Layers of Interoperability	68
	Interoperability Standards	68
	Why Interoperability Is Hard	69
	HL7 FHIR	70
	RESTful APIs	71
	Structured Data	72
	Use Cases	72
	FHIR Resources	73
	Questionnaire	74
	QuestionnaireResponse	74
	Relationships with Other Resources	77
	Workflow	77
	Coding Schemes	80
	LOINC	80
	SNOMED CT	81
	References	83
8	**Value of Health and Lives**	85
	Death Rates	85
	Value of a Statistical Life (VSL)	85
	Preference Measures	86
	QALY Model	87
	Load Model	89
	A Worked Example	90
	Discussion	95
	References	95
II	**Measures**	
9	**Patient-Reported Measures**	99
	Core Outcome Sets	99
	Taxonomy	99
	Patient and Staff-Reported	100
	PROMs Domains	101
	PREMs Domains	101
	Option Sets	101
	Table	102
	Quality of Life	103
	Individual Care	103
	Care Provided	105
	Provider Culture	105

		Innovation	105
		References	110
10	**Patient Experience**		111
	Background		111
	Development		112
		Devising Items	112
		Scoring	114
		Readability	115
	Case Study		115
		Distribution	116
		Validation	117
	Service Integration		119
	Friends and Family Test		121
	References		122
11	**Health Status**		125
	Background		125
		SF-36 and SF-12	126
		EQ-5D	127
		howRu Health Status Measure	129
	Case Study 1		131
		Method	131
		Distribution of Scores	131
		Internal Structure	132
		Validity	133
	Case Study 2		133
		Results	134
	Correlations		137
	Comparisons		138
	Conclusions		139
	References		139
12	**Wellbeing**		141
	Background		141
	Subjective Wellbeing		141
		ONS4	142
		PWS	143
	EQ Health and Wellbeing		144
	Mental Health		144
		WEMWBS	145
		ReQoL	145
		Comparisons	146
	References		148

13	**Patient-Centred Care**	149
	Patient-Centered Care	149
	Self-efficacy	149
	Supported Self-management	150
	Measures	151
	Case Study	154
	Comparison of Measures	155
	Shared Decision-Making	155
	CollaboRATE	157
	Shared Decisions	157
	References	158
14	**Individualised Measures**	159
	Background	159
	Individualised Measures	160
	MYCaW	160
	Person-Specific Outcome	161
	Comparisons	163
	Conclusions	163
	References	164
15	**How People Live**	165
	Social Determinants of Health	165
	Health Index for England	165
	Social Determinants Measure	166
	Loneliness and Social Contact	168
	Loneliness Measures	168
	Social Contact	169
	Loneliness	170
	Case Study—Social Contact	171
	Discussion	174
	Length and Readability	174
	References	175
16	**Innovation Evaluation**	177
	Innovation	177
	Measures	178
	Innovation Readiness	179
	Digital Confidence	181
	Innovation Process	182
	Product Satisfaction	183
	Behaviour Change	184
	Training	185
	Digital Competence	187

	Product Confidence	187
	Case Study—Digital Readiness in General Practice	188
	Comparison of Measures	189
	Conclusions	190
	References	190
17	**Staff-Reported Measures**	193
	Background	193
	Quality of Life	194
	Individual Care	194
	Care Provided	194
	Provider Culture	195
	Innovation	196
	References	200
18	**Proxies, Caregivers and Care Home Residents**	201
	Proxies	201
	Caregivers	201
	Case Study	202
	Care Home Residents	204
	References	204
Appendix		207
Index		219

About the Author

Tim Benson has spent most of his career in healthcare, focusing on healthcare computing. He originally trained as a mechanical engineer at the University of Nottingham, where he designed built and tested one of the first hovercraft built outside the aerospace industry.

He joined the NHS in 1974 to lead the evaluation of new computer systems being introduced at the Charing Cross Hospital in London. There he met some of the pioneers of healthcare outcome measures and saw their potential.

In 1980, he established one of the first GP computer suppliers, which developed problem-oriented patient records for use in the consulting room and the Read Codes, which led later to SNOMED CT. From about 1990, he focused on health interoperability, HL7 and later FHIR.

In the mid-2000s, he began a project to develop a short generic health outcome measure. This was followed by a patient experience and other measures, leading to founding R-Outcomes Ltd. more work on PROMs and PREMs and this book.

Part I
Principles

Why PROMs and PREMs Matter?

Introduction

Health care systems aim to reduce the burden of illness, injury and disability, and improve the health and functioning of the people they serve [1]. There is broad consensus that health care provision should be:

- *Safe*—avoid harm to patients from care intended to help them.
- *Effective*—avoiding underuse and overuse of services by providing them to all who could benefit and not to those unlikely to benefit, based on scientific evidence.
- *Patient-centred*—provide care that takes full account of individual patient preferences, needs and values.
- *Timely*—minimise waits and delays for care recipients and providers.
- *Efficient*—avoid all avoidable waste.
- *Equitable*—provide top quality care to all.

Sadly, we seldom measure how safe, effective, patient-centred, efficient, or equitable most health services really are. Rather, we measure how much work they do and when, but not the amount of benefit they provide. Yet, you cannot improve what you do not measure.

Health services generate vast amounts of data, which grows exponentially. To put this in perspective, the sum of all the words ever spoken by human beings comes to about 5 exabytes. An exabyte is enormous; it is 10^9 gigabytes (10,000,000,000 GB). Yet, health data is already bigger than this although little of this data helps us know how patients are doing.

The Quality Chasm

Around the turn of the century, the US Institute of Medicine (IoM) identified a gap in quality between what was delivered and what was needed. They called it a chasm [1]. An earlier report, *To Err is Human,* showed that healthcare systems lacked the environment, processes, and capabilities to ensure that health care was safe, effective, or equitable [2]. In the USA alone, about 100,000 people were dying each year because of basic errors due to:

1. The growing complexity of science and technology
2. The increase in chronic conditions
3. Poorly organised delivery systems
4. Constraints on exploiting information technology.

Healthcare service lack any effective feedback mechanism to show how well the system is working [3]. Waste is enormous. The IoM has estimated annual waste in US health care at $765 billion [4], made up of:(1) Unnecessary services ($210 billion) (2) Inefficiency ($130 billion) (3) Excess administrative costs ($190 billion) (4) Prices that are too high ($105 billion) (5) Missing prevention opportunities ($55 billion) (6) Fraud ($75 billion).

Case and Deaton in *Deaths of Despair and the Future of Capitalism*, writing before the COVID pandemic, demonstrate that for many people things have progressed from bad to worse [5].

Quality Measures

Writing in the mid-1960s, Avedis Donabedian identified three types of information relevant to healthcare quality: structure, process, and outcome [6]:

Structure covers the context of care. It includes the number, skills and relationships of staff, the equipment available, buildings used and financial resources available. This limits what the system can achieve.

Process is the activities that people do to provide healthcare. This includes the number and appropriateness of diagnoses, procedures, and treatments done.

Outcome is the impact on patients and populations, including changes in health status, prognosis, behaviour, knowledge, experience, and satisfaction. Ultimately this is what matters to patients and their families. Outcome measurement is not easy, because many outcomes depend on case-mix—what is the matter with the patient—and other outcomes may not show until many years later.

Donabedian's framework scales from the smallest clinic to whole regions. It is often drawn with arrows from structure to process and from process to outcome. But, while good structure can enable process and process can enable outcome, there is no certainty. It is complex.

Investments in structure may or may not help deliver better process or outcomes. Some activities (process) do more harm than good. Outcomes are impacted by inequalities and social determinants of health [7], and by unwarranted variation in clinical practice [8].

What Do Health Care Systems Produce?

A fundamental question is how to define what health care systems produce. What is produced for the money spent? Sometimes this is straightforward, such as setting a broken bone. But it is often more complicated. For example, consider a patient with both insulin-dependent diabetes and COPD (chronic obstructive airways disease). Using steroids to treat a COPD exacerbation may raise blood glucose and exacerbate diabetes-related problems. Treatment for one condition may make others worse.

One approach is to say that the product of health care is the sum of the set of goods and services provided to each individual patient, including tests, treatment, and other services, all of which can be priced or costed. Activity, and hence cost data, can come from billing systems if every item of service is tracked. Case-mix measures such as Diagnosis Related Groups (DRGs) are used to group patients with broadly similar costs, processes, and outcomes.

DRGs were conceived as a research tool to help answer questions such as: "Why do some patients stay in hospital longer and have more tests than others [9]?" DRGs were later co-opted for use as a basis for payment. The idea was that each DRG would constrain the expected care and services required for each class of patient, against which actual care patterns can be compared. This attention would reduce unwarranted variation. Other countries have also adopted the DRG approach. In the NHS they are called Health Related Groups (HRGs).

Resource allocation by DRG was an improvement on the previous approach of controlling expenditure by giving each functional department (wards, laboratories, theatres, etc.) their own budget. Rigid budgets created perverse incentives. Some people did not do tests that were needed or did tests that are not needed, just to meet budget targets.

However, the DRG approach led to rapid price inflation because providers found extra conditions that put patients into higher priced categories (DRG inflation). Also, DRGs are essentially a classification of health care activities (process) and are silent about outcome.

Personalised Care

The Triple Aim

In 1997, Don Berwick wrote:

> The ultimate measure by which to judge the quality of a medical effort is whether it helps patients (and their families) as they see it. Anything done in healthcare that does not help a patient or their family is, by definition, waste [3].

He later expanded this into the *Triple Aim*—care, health and cost—which became the organising framework for the US National Quality Strategy [10].

- Improve the experience of care and engage patients to play an active role in their care to improve safety and outcomes.
- Improve the health of populations, prevent, and manage long-term conditions.
- Reduce per capita costs of health care, reduce resource use and readmissions and accept greater risk.

Some have also added a fourth aim (Quadruple Aim), to improve the satisfaction of healthcare professionals, reduce staff burden and burnout [11].

Person-centred care

The aim of person-centred care is to improve people's health and wellbeing, to join up care in local communities, and to reduce pressure on healthcare services. It is expected to help people with multiple physical and mental health conditions to make decisions about managing their health, so they can live the life they want to live, based on what matters to them.

NHS England defines personalised care, which means the same as person-centred care, as follows [12]:

> Personalised care means people have choice and control over the way their care is planned and delivered. It is based on 'what matters' to them and their individual strengths and needs.
>
> Personalised care takes a whole-system approach, integrating services around the person including health, social care, public health and wider services. It provides an all-age approach from conception right through to end of life, encompassing both mental and physical health and recognises the role and voice of carers. It recognises the contribution of communities and the voluntary and community sector to support people and build resilience.

The key components include [13]:

- Shared decision-making so people understand the benefits, risks and consequences of different options and make fully informed decisions.
- Personalised care and support planning so people have a plan with a single named coordinator to address their needs.
- Enabling choice of healthcare provider.

- Social prescribing to link to local and community support services and to address non-medical determinants of heath.
- Supported self-management to improve people's knowledge, skills and confidence to look after their own long-term conditions, and to seek help when appropriate.
- Personal health budgets to support a person's identified health and wellbeing needs.

The intention is that personalised care becomes the new normal.

PROMs and PREMs

Patient-reported outcome measures (PROMs) and patient-reported experience measures (PREMs) support the Triple and Quadruple aims and person-centred care.

PROMs and PREMs are questionnaires, used to measure respondents' perceptions of the outcome and experience of health and care services. In our definitions we use the term *person-reported* because similar measures can be completed by patients, health care staff and unpaid carers (caregivers).

The Institute of Medicine has recommended that the term *patient* be replaced be *person*, because the term patient implies that a person under active management by a specific provider, which is too restrictive [14]. Our use also includes proxies, staff and caregivers.

PROMs

Person-reported outcome measures (PROMs) measure people's perception of their own situation. PROMs are personal history, which may be clinically valuable. PROMs support communication between patients and healthcare professionals, and inform service improvement, health policy, health technology evaluation and pharmaceutics labelling claims. PROMs can offer large benefits to patients and society, but current use is fragmented and suboptimal [15].

To track individual patients over time, and/or use the results in clinical decisions, you need to identify the patient in some way. This can be done in several ways but brings in issues of personal privacy and information governance that must be dealt with at the start.

Barriers hindering the use of PROMs in routine care are discussed in Chaps. 4 and 5.

PREMs

Person-reported experience measures (PREMs) measure respondent's perception of services provided. PREMs are usually completed anonymously as people are often reluctant to criticise those they depend on, for fear of reprisals. Individuals may choose to identify themselves in PREMs, but the default is not to.

We need to distinguish between three types of PROMs and PREMs—condition-specific, generic, and individualised.

Condition-specific

Condition-specific measures apply to one condition only. Thousands of condition-specific measures have been developed, mainly supported by the pharmaceutical industry, which needs evidence from randomised clinical trials to justify claims to drug regulators before products can be licensed.

However, more than 70% of health and care expenditure is for people living with three or more conditions, and condition-specific PROMs apply to one only. Multiple conditions limit their use of as part of routine health and care processes. Similar constraints apply to treatment-specific measures.

Generic

Generic measures apply to all types of persons, treatments, and conditions; they are based on the idea that most people have similar needs and hopes. People look for good health and well-being, excellent service, supportive communities and organisations, care and innovations that work for them.

Generic measures are independent of patients' conditions or services received. However, many generic measures are less sensitive than condition-specific measures, but have advantages in many parts of health and care, such as when people have multiple conditions. Most measures described in this book are generic.

Individualised

Individualised measures focus on what people say are their most important issues at the time, and measure progress for these issues. Individualised measures are usually used alongside generic measures. They are discussed further in Chap. 14.

Criteria

Similar criteria apply to all types of PROMs and PREMs. These include brevity, clarity, relevance, genericity, multi-modal, multi-attribute, responsiveness, and psychometric properties. These are briefly discussed below:

Brevity

Keeping instruments as short as possible means that they are quick to use by patients, or proxies if patients are too ill to complete it themselves.

Word count is a measure of brevity.

Clarity

Wording should be unambiguous and meaningful to respondents. The instrument must be readily understood by vulnerable people and translated accurately into other languages.

Readability (see Chap. 3) is a measure of clarity.

Relevance

Instruments should be suitable for frequent and repeated use. Some measures are more responsive to treatment than others. Some are likely to fluctuate, while others remain more stable.

Response rate is a way to measure acceptability and relevance.

Generic

Generic instruments are applicable without change across all patient categories and care settings, including primary, secondary, community, emergency, domiciliary and social care. A generic measure can be used with any combination of patients' diagnoses and treatment.

Multi-modal

Methods of data collection (modalities) include paper, touchscreen devices (such as kiosks, smartphones, and tablets), web browsers and telephones, including automated interactive voice response (IVR) systems.

Multi-attribute

Instruments need to cover the most important dimensions (attributes) of outcomes and experience, as identified by potential users and in the literature.

Responsiveness

Instruments should be sensitive to change and only include items under the day-to-day control of local staff and management. Things should usually be excluded that cannot be changed at local level, such as location, transport, car-parking, payments, regulations, and legislation.

Psychometric properties

Instruments need to demonstrate validity and good psychometric properties, including response distribution (including ceiling and floor effects) and internal consistency.

A *ceiling effect* is found when people choose the top (best) option, so the measure is not able to detect any further improvement. A *floor effect* is when people choose the bottom (worst) option, so further deterioration cannot be detected. Ceiling and floor effects are most important in before measures, when questionnaires are used to measure change before and after an intervention. They can apply to specific items or to a whole measure.

Lessons

Lessons on what does and does not work when implementing PROMs and PREMs include:

1. Those who commission surveys need to communicate a clear vision of the purpose and how the results will be used.
2. People will complete surveys if asked to do so nicely, ideally face to face, and if the survey is not too burdensome. Expect a low response rate if either is not true.
3. Time spent on planning what questions to ask and how best to do it is well spent.
4. Health and care are complex—multiple measures are usually needed.
5. Some measures improve with good care, but some do not; these may provide important contextual information.
6. Point-in-time measures can be anonymous. These may be useful for accountability and quality improvement.
7. To show individual progress, you need some sort of identifier. Use identifiers that are easy to use for the patient and acceptable to information governance professionals.
8. Clinical decision-makers need individual results when tailoring care and treatment.
9. Information governance is more complicated when individual results are shared.
10. Data collection is easier when it is part of routine work (the way we do things here), not an optional extra.
11. Different users have different likes and needs when it comes to reviewing results. For some it is a large part of their job, but not for others. Some like detailed tables, others like charts.
12. At every stage, be crystal clear about who does what, when, where, how, and why.

Conclusions

Traditionally, the PROMs agenda was driven by researchers and service payers. It did not focus on improving the quality of care from the patients' perspective [15]. This is now changing, in part due to increased focus on personalised care. PROMs and PREMs can be used at multiple levels within the health care system:

- Whole health systems assess performance and assessing value for money.
- Healthcare providers monitor performance, quality improvement and benchmarking against comparable units.
- Clinical trials measure treatment outcomes and screen eligibility.

- Clinical practice includes structured history taking, to monitor progress and to aid diagnosis and treatment.
- Patients need to communicate with clinicians—to help in shared decision making about choice of treatment or provider.

PROMs can help narrow the gap between clinician's and patient's view of reality and to tailor treatment to meet the patient's preferences and needs. PROMs let patients tell their clinicians about what happens outside the clinical encounter, such as symptoms, response to treatment, unwanted side effects and their needs and wants. They can raise clinicians' awareness of patients' problems and prompt discussion and action [16].

However, research on attempts to embed routine measurement of PROMs into routine practice have revealed a wide range of behavioral, technical, social, cultural, legal and logistical barriers to successful adoption. These are discussed in Chaps. 4 and 5. First we briefly consider the history of PROMs and PREMs up to 2010.

References

1. Institute of Medicine. Crossing the quality chasm: a new health system for the 21st century. Washington: National Academy Press; 2001.
2. Institute of Medicine. To err is human: building a safer health system. Washington: National Academy Press; 2000.
3. Berwick D. Medical associations: guilds or leaders—either play the role of victim or actively work to improve healthcare systems. BMJ. 1997;314:1564.
4. Institute of Medicine. Best care at lower cost: the path to a continuously learning healthcare in America. Washington: National Academy Press; 2013.
5. Case A, Deaton A. Deaths of despair and the future of capitalism. Princeton University Press; 2020.
6. Donabedian A. Evaluating the quality of medical care. Millbank Memorial Fund Quarterly. 1966;44(3):166–203.
7. Marmot M. The health gap: the challenge of an unequal world. London: Bloomsbury; 2015.
8. Wennberg J. Tracking medicine: a researcher's quest to understand health care. Oxford University Press; 2010.
9. Fetter R, Shin Y, Freeman J, et al. Case mix definition by diagnosis-related groups. Med Care. 1980;18(2 Suppl) iii:1–53.
10. Berwick D, Nolan T, Whittington J. The triple aim: care, health, and cost. Health Aff. 2008;27(3):759–69.
11. Sikka R, Morath JM, Leape L. The quadruple aim: care, health, cost and meaning in work. BMJ Qual Saf. 2015;24:608–10.
12. NHS England. The NHS long term plan. 2019. https://www.longtermplan.nhs.uk/wpcontent/uploads/2019/01/nhs-long-term-plan.pdf
13. NHS England. Universal personalised care: implementing the comprehensive model. 2019. https://www.england.nhs.uk/personalisedcare/
14. Institute of Medicine. Building data capacity for patient-centered outcomes research: interim report 1—Looking ahead at data needs. Washington, DC: The National Academies Press; 2021.

15. Calvert M, Kyte D, Price G, et al. Maximising the impact of patient reported outcome assessment for patients and society. BMJ. 2019;364:k5267.
16. Greenhalgh J, Gooding K, Gibbons E, et al. How do patient reported outcome measures (PROMs) support clinician-patient communication and patient care? A realist synthesis. J Patient-Rep Outcomes. 2018;2(1):1–28.

History 2

Early Pioneers

Outcome measure use in health care can be traced back to the Scottish Enlightenment of the 18th Century. Each year the Edinburgh Infirmary published statistics on the condition of patients as they left the hospital. Patients were reported as *cured, relieved, incurable, died* or *dismissed by desire or for irregularities* [1].

These ideas were taken up many years later by Florence Nightingale following her return from the Crimean War, who set up a scheme at St Thomas' Hospital London in which patients were classified on discharge. She introduced a simple classification of health outcomes in the 1860s and argued that this be widely adopted:

> I am fain to sum up with an urgent appeal for adopting this or some uniform system for publishing the statistical records of hospitals. There is a growing conviction that in all hospitals, even those which are best conducted, there is a great and unnecessary waste of life. In attempting to arrive at the truth, I have applied everywhere for information, but in scarcely an instance have I been able to obtain hospital records fit for any purpose of comparison. If they could be obtained, they would enable us to decide many other questions beside the ones alluded to. They would show subscribers how their money was being spent, what amount of good was really being done with it, or whether their money was not doing mischief rather than good [2].

Her system was implemented in several teaching hospitals and continued for more than 100 years, until it was replaced by the national Hospital Activity Analysis scheme (HAA) [3]. HAA provided detailed data on hospital activity, but nothing about whether patients received any benefit.

In the USA before World War I, surgeon Ernest Codman promoted his *End Results* system, which was based on the idea that surgeons should be open and transparent about the outcomes of treatment, including failures as well as successes. For advocating such openness, he paid a heavy price; he was ostracised by his colleagues and forced to stand down as chair of the Boston Surgical Society [4].

The Apgar Score

The Apgar score is a good but surprisingly rare example of a clinically-specific measure that has stood the test of time. The Apgar score is used worldwide to evaluate the health of new-born babies [5]. See Fig. 2.1.

The score was developed in 1952 by Virginia Apgar, an anaesthetist, not a midwife nor an obstetrician. Each baby is scored on five objective findings: appearance, pulse, grimace, activity and respiration (these form a *backronym* for Apgar).

The test is done at 1 and 5 min after birth and may be repeated later if results are low. The score is calculated by adding the scores 0, 1 or 2 (with 2 being the best score) for each dimension, giving a range from 0 (5 × 0) to 10 (5 × 2). A score of 7 or above is normal, 4 to 6 is fairly low and 3 or below is critically low, requiring immediate intervention. In her original paper, Apgar described a tenfold difference in the average perinatal mortality rates between each group defined by these thresholds [5].

The Apgar score focuses attention on five dimensions that drive clinical decisions. It uses objective categories for each dimension and a standard scoring system to arrive at an overall score. It is short and quick to use in the confusion of a delivery room. Critically, inter-rater reliability is far higher than the neonatal clinical judgements used previously (see Chap. 5 for a discussion as to why this is the case).

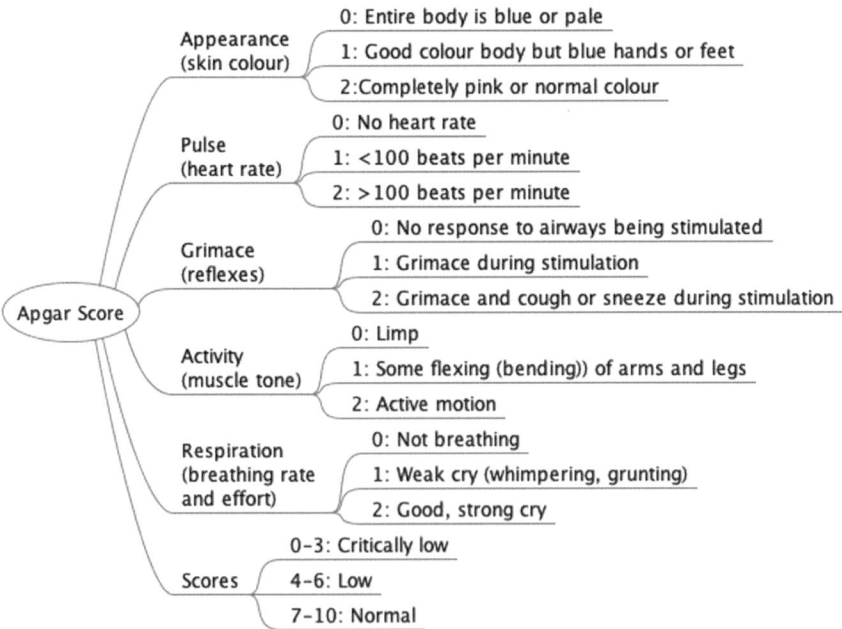

Fig. 2.1 Apgar Score including scoring scheme

At the time that the Apgar score was developed, the death rate for babies in the USA was more than 30 per 1,000. Today, that figure is about 2 per 1,000.

Atul Gawande wrote:

> The Apgar score changed everything. It was practical and easy to calculate, and it gave clinicians at the bedside immediate feedback on how effective their care was. In the rest of medicine we are used to measuring dozens of specific things: blood counts, electrolyte levels, heart rates, viral titres. But we have no routine measure that puts the data together to grade how the patient as a whole is faring. We have only an impression of how we're performing—and sometimes not even that [6].

Part of the vision for using PROMs and PREMs is to help clinicians and mangers understand how they are performing.

PROMs

Before 1980

In the period after World War II, there was widespread optimism about scientific progress, exemplified by the triumph of antibiotics, space travel and information technology. However, it was recognised increasingly that much of what was done in healthcare was neither efficient nor effective [7].

Tudor Hart's Inverse Care Law showed that the availability of good healthcare varied inversely with the need for it in the population served [8]. Fifty years' later these inequalities persist. Socially disadvantaged people still receive less and poorer quality care despite having greatest needs [9].

Sir Colin Dollery, a founding father of clinical pharmacology, wrote:

> The least satisfactory part of the application of science to medicine has been in the evaluation of diagnostic and therapeutic procedures as they are generally used in the process of medical care. The medical profession has been too ready to believe that each new discovery is a breakthrough which can be adopted universally based on limited studies in highly selected patients. There are too few well designed studies of the real benefits and costs of new and old methods of care. Without such studies better allocation of resources is impossible, and the alternative is a crude form of rationing based largely on existing patterns [10].

In 1966, President Johnson set a national goal of *the highest level of health attainable for every person* and the need for comprehensive planning of health service provision. In response, Fanshel and Bush [11] proposed a health status index, comprising an index of well-being and prognosis. The index of well-being was defined using a classification of levels on a continuum of function/dysfunction, scored on a scale from 0 (absolute dysfunction or death) to 1 (100% function). Prognosis was defined as the transitional probability of change in functional state with time, but this has proved difficult to measure.

In Canada, Torrance [12] used a similar function/dysfunction scale and estimated the utility of different states for specific conditions using two different methods (standard gamble and time trade-off)—see also Chap. 8.

In England, Culyer, Lavers and Williams developed a conceptual framework of indicators of health status, need and effectiveness, but did not develop scales of valuation for health states [13]. Rosser and Watts developed a classification of disability and distress, which they used to measure the output of a London hospital [14]. This involved the classification of all patients on admission, discharge and out-patient follow-up appointment following discharge and on the first and last day of a one-month study. Their disability and distress classification separated physical function from mental well-being. Initially, Rosser used a scale of illness based on the awards made by the courts to victims of accidents. Her original aim was to specify minimal data requirements that could be collected routinely for all patients [15]. Later she used methods of magnitude estimation to develop a different scale of illness, using long structured interviews with 70 patients [16].

My own experience with outcome measures started in 1976 when I met Rachel Rosser, while leading the Computer Evaluation Unit at the Charing Cross Hospital in London. We used a mixed methods approach to evaluate the computer project in the hospital but without the outcomes dimension. The Department of Health extended our remit to do this.

I used Rosser and Watts' classification of disability and distress, which had eight disability classes and four distress classes, and asked ward nurses to rate the patients on six wards every day for three months. At this time, the personal computer had not yet been invented and measures were staff-reported.

At the start, I set up several group sessions in which several nurses rated all the patients on each ward. To my surprise, inter-rater agreement was low. I then held group meetings of the raters to discuss what they should have recorded. There a high level of consensus was reached. Subsequently I repeated the inter-rater agreement studies and found excellent agreement. This led to important conclusions [17]. The English language is ambiguous, and people interpret the same terms in different ways. This can be sorted by training.

There are two main ways to train people. Either rely on universal teaching, such as is provided to primary school children, or arrange special training sessions, which is not practical for patients. A simple example will make the point. Almost everyone knows the difference between the pink and purple because they are taught at primary school, but fewer know the difference between magenta (purplish-red) and cyan (greenish-blue), because these are not. (Magenta, cyan and yellow are the three colours used in most colour printers).

This study recorded nearly 4,000 ratings by staff of patients and demonstrated the practicality of measuring health status routinely in a large NHS hospital. Acceptable methods of data collection were developed, including direct entry into patients' nursing records and onto forms on which patient names had already been entered.

Analytic techniques included the development of patient profiles, showing patient's progress day-to-day and ward profiles showing the changes in the mean or median health status of all patients on each ward. A hospital-wide nursing information system was proposed, which would have used patient's health status information to guide the allocation of nursing resources on a day-to-day basis. This was not pursued and the project closed in 1980. I went to work on GP computing [18] and health interoperability [19], before returning to outcome measurement twenty-five years later.

1980s

Important foundations were laid for future developments during the 1980s. These include the development of the concepts of quality adjusted life years (QALYs) and patient-reported outcome measures.

QALYs

The term Quality Adjusted Life Year (QALY) was first proposed in the 1970s [20] and began to be used widely during the 1980s. The QALY is a simple idea intuitively, but remains controversial for reasons explored in Chap. 8. Perfect health is valued at one and dead is valued as zero. If we only have two states (alive and dead), the sum over time is equivalent to life expectancy. Morbidity is introduced by giving ill patients a value less than one, so adding quality-adjustment to life years.

Additional complexity may be introduced by allowing states worse than dead to account for assisted dying and discounting future states. However, achieving a population consensus on the values of health states relative to the zero to one continuum has proven to be unexpectedly hard.

The QALY concept was boosted by the publication of a short but influential review of coronary-artery bypass grafts (CABG) [21], and the first textbook to cover QALYs in detail [22].

Patient-Reported Outcomes

Increased recognition that clinical outcomes did not always reflect what mattered most to patients or their families led to increased interest in patient-reported outcomes.

In one example, a study of treatment for 75 patients with high blood pressure found that all of the doctors thought that medication led to improvement, as objectively demonstrated by reduced blood pressure, but less than half of patients and only a single relative thought it had helped. Most relatives classified the adverse changes as moderate or severe. These deteriorations were attributed to preoccupation with sickness, decline in energy, general and sexual activity, and irritability—none of which leave objectively measurable clinical signs [23].

1990s

Concerns about differences between clinicians' and patients' perceptions of outcome led to patient-reported outcomes being mandated in applications for approval by medicines regulators such as the FDA (Food and Drug Administration).

Two important HRQL measures were published: SF-36 and EQ-5D [24]. These are described in more detail in Chap. 11, Health Status.

Pharmaco-Economics

Political interest in patient-reported outcomes increased during the 1990s, especially in relation to drug regulation and approval. Pharmaceutical companies realised that to get new drugs approved they needed to provide evidence of cost-effectiveness. The way this happened differed in different countries.

In the UK the National Institute for Health and Clinical Excellence (NICE) was established in 1999 with the aim to create consistent guidelines and end rationing of treatment by post code. Technology Assessments (TAs) are based on the core metric of Incremental Cost-Effectiveness Ratio (ICER), expressed in terms of cost per QALY [25]. This needs a standard way of measuring QALYs using generic preference-based measures of health, such as EQ-5D or SF-6D.

Academic Societies

Two international multi-disciplinary academic societies, ISOQOL and ISPOR were also founded during this period.

ISOQOL (International Society for Quality of Life Research) focuses on health-related quality of life research (HRQL), including the patients' voice. ISOQOL was founded in 1994 and has about 1,200 members, many of whom are health psychologists. Its main publications are *Quality of Life Research journal (QLR)* and *Journal of Patient-Reported Outcomes (JPRO)*.

ISPOR (International Society for Pharmaco-economics and Outcomes Research) has a mission to improve decision-making for health globally. ISPOR was founded in 1995 and mainly attracts health economists and people in the pharmaceutical industry; it has more than 20,000 members. Its main publication is *Value in Health*.

2000s

The early years of the 21st Century were a period of optimism for advocates of PROMs and PREMs. Politicians listened to arguments that patients' views were important.

In the USA, the Institute of Health Improvement defined the Triple Aim, which aims to: (1) improve the quality of care, (2) improve the health of populations and (3) reduce per capita costs of health care [26]. These three aspects are related in complex ways but all are important. Three preconditions are: (1) specifying a population of concern, not individual patients, (2) impose policy constraints to ensure equality, (3) and have an effective integrator to ensure that all three aims are prioritised.

The Triple Aim has an implicit assumption that organisations will measure PROMs and PREMs as well as costs (see Chap. 1).

In the UK, a major government report (*High Quality Care for All*) defined quality in terms of patient safety, patient experience and effectiveness. Experience and effectiveness would be measured using PREMs and PROMs. All hospitals were required to publish annual quality reports and greater transparency would encourage staff to improve their own performance [27].

Since April 2009 the NHS in England has required all patients having four procedures, including hip and knee replacement surgery, to complete a pair of PROMs before the operation and after their recovery [28]. This scheme continues but has not expanded. (See also Chap. 11).

Routine measurement of PROMs and PREMs has proved to be harder in practice than many people expected. The reasons are explored in Chapter 4 (Why PROMs are hard: people) and Chapter 5 (Noise and complexity).

References

1. Risse GB. Hospital life in enlightenment Scotland. Cambridge University Press; 1986. p. 43–59.
2. Nightingale F. Notes on hospitals. 3rd ed. London: Longman, Green, Longman, Roberts and Green; 1863.
3. Rosser R. A history of the development of health indicators. In: Teeling Smith G, editor. Measuring the social benefits of medicine. London: Office of Health Economics; 1983. p. 50–62.
4. Neuhauser D. Ernest Amory Codman MD. BMJ Qual Saf. 2002;11:104–5.
5. Apgar V. A proposal for a new method of evaluation of the newborn infant. Curr Res Anaesth Analg. 1953;32(4):250–9.
6. Gawande A. Better: a surgeon's notes on performance. London: Profile Books; 2007. p. 190.
7. Cochrane A. Effectiveness and efficiency; random reflections on health services. London: Nuffield Provincial Hospitals Trust; 1972.
8. Tudor HL. The inverse care law. Lancet. 1971;297:405–12.
9. Cookson R, Doran T, Asaria M, et al. The inverse care law re-examined: a global perspective. Lancet. 2021;397:828–38.
10. Dollery C. The end of an age of optimism: medical science in retrospect and prospect. London: Nuffield Provincial Hospitals Trust; 1978.
11. Fanshel S, Bush J. A health status index and its application to health services outcomes. Oper Res. 1970;18:1021–66.
12. Torrance G, Thomas W, Sackett D. A utility maximization model for evaluation of health care programs. Health Serv Res. 1972;7:118–33.
13. Culyer A, Lavers R, Williams A. Social indicators: health. Soc Trends. 1971; 2:31-42.
14. Rosser R, Watts V. The measurement of hospital output. Int J Epidemiol. 1972;1:361–8.
15. Rosser R. A health index and output measure. In: Walker S, Rosser R, editors. Quality of life assessment: key issues in the 1990s. Dordrecht: Springer; 1993. https://doi.org/10.1007/978-94-011-2988-6_7

16. Rosser R, Kind P. A scale of valuations of states of illness: is there a social consensus? Int J Epidemiol. 1978;7:347–58.
17. Benson T. Classification of disability and distress by ward nurses: a reliability study. Int J Epidemiol. 1978;7:359–61.
18. Benson T. Why general practitioners use computers and hospital doctors do not—Part 1: incentives and Part 2: scalability. BMJ. 2002;325:1086–93.
19. Benson T, Grieve G. Principles of health interoperability FHIR HL7 and SNOMED CT. 4th ed. London: Springer; 2021.
20. Stason M, Weinstein W. Foundations of cost-effectiveness analysis for health and medical practices. NEJM. 1977;296(13):716–21.
21. Williams A. Economics of coronary artery bypass grafting. BMJ. 1985;291:326–9.
22. Drummond M, Stoddart G, Torrance G. Methods for the economic evaluation of health care programmes. Oxford University Press; 1987.
23. Jachuk SJ, Brierley H, Jachuk S, Willcox P. The effect of hypotensive drugs on the quality of life. JRCGP. 1982;32:103–5.
24. Brazier J, Ratcliffe J, Salomon JA, Tsuchiya A. Measuring and valuing health benefits for economic evaluation. 2nd ed. Oxford University Press; 2016.
25. Williams A. What could be nicer than NICE. London: Office of Health Economics; 2004.
26. Berwick D, Nolan T, Whittington J. The Triple Aim: care, health and cost. Health Aff. 2008;27(3):759–69.
27. Darzi A. High quality care for all: NHS next stage review final report. Stationery Office; 2008.
28. Devlin N, Appleby J. Getting the most out of PROMs: putting health outcomes at the heart of NHS decision-making. London: The Kings Fund; 2010.

Terms 3

Descriptive Framework

All measures have a descriptive framework (the questions) and a scoring scheme.

The term descriptive framework is what the respondent sees. It can apply to a whole questionnaire or to individual measures.

Questionnaire

A *questionnaire* is an instrument, presented on a screen or paper, consisting of a series of questions to gather information from respondents. The term *survey* is often used as a synonym for questionnaire, but survey also has a broader meaning covering the whole process of designing, collecting, analysing and reporting a study.

PROMs and PREMs have been developed by many different groups. In general, different tools do not work well together. Caution is needed when using measures from different development groups in the same questionnaire. There are often big differences between measures in both the descriptive framework and the scoring scheme.

Typically, PROMs and PREMs questionnaires include one or more validated measures plus demographic data.

Demographics

Demographic data provide appropriate context. It usually makes sense to follow local custom and use the norm where you are working. However, consider how the information will be used and who needs to know each data item. Even supposedly simple items like gender can give rise to long debates about the number of options needed.

Demographic data create problems with respect to privacy and information governance. Privacy laws require that identifiable data be handled in ways that meet the spirit and letter of the regulations. In practice, this means that we must be careful with any data that could allow the respondent to be identified; all items of demographic data must be fully justified. It is often better to allow an item to be optional rather than add additional boxes for "I would rather not say" or "I do not know".

If in doubt, leave it out. If you do need an item, choose the simplest set of options that meet the need and try to make all groups the same size. For example, we often need to know age group. Deciles are a simple way of collecting this, but some organizations like to use different age thresholds, such as 16, 18, 21, 25 and so on, for obscure or historical reasons.

Role

Always be clear about four separate human roles: *requester*, *respondent*, *subject* and *data enterer*. These may or may not be the same person. Consider two simple use cases.

1. Anna is sent an email message by a healthcare provider, which contains a URL link to a questionnaire; she completes the online questionnaire herself. In this case the *requester* is the provider and Anna is *respondent*, *subject* and *data enterer*.
2. Simon (the subject) attends Daisy's clinic with his daughter Rose. Simon has Alzheimer's Disease and cannot complete a questionnaire himself. Daisy (*requester*) asks them to complete a short questionnaire. Daisy reads out the questions, which Rose (*respondent*) answers verbally, acting as a proxy for Simon (*subject*). The data is entered immediately into the computer questionnaire by Daisy (*data enterer*).

Measure

Measure refers to a specific set of items and options, which address some construct of interest. A construct is any idea or theory containing various conceptual elements, typically considered to be subjective.

Each measure usually has a name, an introductory text or instructions (often called a preamble), a set of items (see below) and response options. Together these are the measure's descriptive framework.

Domain is sometimes used as a synonym for measure but may be broader. *Dimension* is also sometimes used as a synonym for measure but is usually narrower. Dimension may also be used as a synonym for item.

Item

Items are the individual questions asked. Items may be thought of as the elements of a construct. Each item is a single question. It usually has a text label and a set of response *options*. Item wording may be positive or negative. A measure may contain any number of items.

For reasons explained in Chaps. 4 and 5, people are not always logical in their assessments. For example, more people would agree to have an operation with 90% chance of survival than one with 10% chance of death, although logically the odds are identical.

Items and measures may have several labels for different tasks:

1. Text—what the respondent sees (e.g., I can get the right help if I need it).
2. Name—self-explanatory out of context (e.g., Access to help).
3. Short name—used in tables where space is limited, often without white space (e.g., GetHelp).

They may also have additional labels for internal computer processing, which are usually invisible to humans. These are often sequences of digits or characters unique within the questionnaire.

Generally, it is good practice to word items positively rather than a negatively, although this cannot always be done due to the inadequacies of languages such as English. For example, English has well understood terms such as pain and discomfort but neither term has a good English antonym (opposite meaning). For example, pain-free is not suitable for a scale, because it is binary—you are, or you are not pain-free; comfort usually refers to a place or feeling, and is not the opposite of discomfort, which usually refers to a person or symptom.

Option

Each item usually has a pre-defined number of defined response *options*. The same option set is normally used for all items in a measure, but there are exceptions. A commonly used set of options is: *Strongly agree*, *Agree*, *Neutral* and *Disagree*. In general, *Strongly agree* and *Agree* imply that people agree with the proposition, and *Neutral* and *Disagree* imply that they do not agree.

Some people like to have a *Strongly disagree* option, but in one-tailed measures this is mainly used by people who like to shout. If a measure is naturally two-tailed, with a symmetrical distribution, then it makes sense for the options to be symmetrical, such as: *Strongly agree*, *Agree*, *Disagree* and *Strongly disagree*.

If an option is used by less than about 3% of a population it is usually only justified if this group has important characteristics that warrant separate identification or action.

The number of options used is a matter of choice and can be anything between 2 and 11. Having many options encourages noise, especially stable pattern noise (see Chap. 5), whereby some people like to use extremities and others prefer to avoid them.

I usually use four well-chosen options. This works well, especially for one-tailed measures. The best option (the ceiling) can be thought of as being as good as it gets. If used appropriately this does not produce a ceiling effect, whereby the measure is unable to detect valuable improvements. A floor effect (the worst option) is more problematic because things can always get worse. In general, if a respondent is at the floor, this calls for action.

I also like to make all questions optional, while encouraging people to complete every item. If people really cannot decide, it often means that there is something wrong with the question. I have found that a separate *don't know* option increases missing values and complicates analysis.

Also avoid multiple-choice options unless there is no alternative. Multiple choice questions produce problems for analysis and people vary in how they use them, creating noise.

Comment

Always try to add at least one free text comment box in every questionnaire, so that people can say exactly what is causing a problem. Any attempt to make an explicit list of all possible problems is likely to be incomplete and too long.

I like to have only one comment box in a questionnaire, which can be signposted at the start. If someone wants to say something they often use the first comment box available, not the one reserved for this comment.

Readability

Poor readability is a self-inflicted error. Survey designers often aim to meet the needs of the people who pay them (such as their manager), rather than those of respondents. Managers are usually well educated and like precise terms, but the average reading age of patients is lower.

The Programme for the International Assessment of Adult Competencies has measured the literary competence of 215,000 people between 16 and 65 years old across 33 countries, allocating them into five levels. Across all OECD countries, about 20% of people were at level 1 or below, with a further 34% at level 2 [1]. Roughly, level 1 equates to a reading age of about 9 (the Gruffalo) and level 2 to a reading age of about 11 (Harry Potter). This suggest that 54% of adults under 65 have a reading age of eleven or less. Reading ability is lower in older people, including most patients. Results from the USA and England are close to OECD averages.

Readability Measures

Text readability is usually measured using tools (listed in order of first publication) such as:

- Flesch Reading Ease Score (FRE) [2];
- Gunning Fog Index [3];
- Standard Measure of Gobbledygook (SMOG) [4];
- Flesch-Kincaid Readability Grade (FKG) [5].

Readability measures work in similar ways, focusing on sentence length and word length. They were not designed for survey items and applicability has been questioned [6]. However, results using different measures are highly correlated [7]. The Fog, SMOG and FKG provide results in terms of the US school grade. US school grade is roughly reading age plus 5. Grade 1 is 6–7 years old; grade 6 is 11–12 years old. Material used by patients, such as surveys and patient information leaflets, should be at grade 5 or lower (reading age 11 or lower) [8, 9].

Most readability measures are available without charge. In this book we use the FKG results from www.readabilityformulas.com.

The way that word count and readability statistics are calculated varies according to which parts of a measure are included. Some measures are stand-alone, while others are used as components in a larger survey. In some measures the options are repeated for each item, in others not. To make comparisons fair, we exclude instructions, framing statements, options and copyright notices.

Some surveys were originally written in one language and translations may misrepresent their performance in their original language.

Translations

Translations create problems because often terms do not have exact translations. For example, if a measure is developed in English, the designer may deliberately use a term with some ambiguity to mean different things. *Quite a lot of pain* could refer to pain intensity or pain continuity (quite a lot of the time). Some languages use distinct terms for each.

Building on earlier work, the PRO Consortium has recommended a 12-step process, which is summarised in Table 3.1 [10]. The full process is required when measures are being used in multi-national clinical trials, and to support drug labelling claims for FDA and other regulators. This can be time-consuming and costly, but a streamlined version may be used for more modest projects.

Key features are that two independent people should translate into the target language and keep a note of all issues met. A third person, with no knowledge of the original should back translate and keep notes. A fourth person should have access to all the working papers and seek to resolve differences, before the draft is pilot tested and further revised.

Scoring Scheme

Analysts and others use the scoring scheme to understand and visualise the data.

Each option can have a *score*, such as 0, 1, 2, etc. Scores may be positive (a high score is good) or negative (a high score is bad). The scoring system should be consistent and easy to understand.

Table 3.1 Summary of PRO Consortium's 12-step translation process

Step #	Step name	Notes
1	Preparation	Plan and recruit
2	Forward translation	Minimum of two independent translations
3	Reconciliation	Make one document with alternatives listed
4	Back translation	At least one backward translation—translator to be blind of source
5	Revision of reconciled forward translation	Evaluate to assess semantic equivalence, list issues, agree revisions and make changes
6	International harmonization	Review for consistency and conceptual equivalence
7	Proofreading	Two independent proof-readers, native from the target language, check for translation and other errors
8	Cognitive interviewing	Pilot tests and cognitive interviews with at least five participants from target population, ideally in person
9	Post-cognitive interview review (analysis/revisions)	Agree any further changes
10	Final review and documentation	Final changes and checks
11	Report	Produce written report
12	Archiving/record-keeping	Keep records

A summary score may be calculated as the sum of the individual item scores for a measure.

Summary score ranges vary enormously for different measures. In this book we include examples with ranges 0–1, 0–10, 0–12, 0–48 and 0–100 (this list is not comprehensive). In some measures a high score is good, in others high is bad. I prefer all scores to point in the same direction with high being desirable and low undesirable.

Weight

Scores are often transformed using different algorithms (*weights*). Commonly used weighting methods include: raw scores, transformed scores, logarithmic scales, normative scales and preference weights.

Raw Scores

Raw scores are simple. An item score is the score for that item, a summary score is the sum of items comprising a measure. For example, a measure may have four items, scored 0, 1, 2, 3 (range 0 to 3), and a summary score with range 0 (4 × 0) to 12 (4 × 3).

Transformed Scores

Transformed scores, for example with a range 0–100, where 0 indicates that all respondents chose the worst options and 100 indicates that they all chose the best options. These are often used for population mean scores. Using the example above, mean item scores are multiplied by 100 and divided by 3; but the mean summary score is multiplied by 100 and divided by 12. This enables item scores and the summary score to be shown on the same scale. These are a type of unweighted scale, retaining a direct arithmetic relationship with the raw scores.

Logarithmic Scales

Logarithmic scales are used where the underlying range is large; they are not widely used in PROMs and PREMs. An example is the decibel (dB)), used in noise measurement. An increase in 10 dB represents ten-fold increase in the power of the noise; a 30 dB increase is a thousand-fold increase in power.

Normative Scales

Normative scales are based on the normal distribution (bell curve), which is widely used in statistics. The SF-36 and SF-12 physical components score (PCS) and mental components score (MCS) are normative scales with mean 50 and standard deviation 10.

A well-known example is the Intelligence Quotient (IQ), where the mean population score is 100 and standard deviation 15. So, if a person is measured as having IQ of 115, their IQ is one standard deviation above the mean. Assuming a normal distribution, IQ of 115 implies that 84% have a lower IQ and 16% have a higher IQ. Normative scales have no upper or lower values.

Preference Weights

Preference weights, where intermediate scores between anchors are given a score derived from population weighting studies. For example, if an intermediate score is weighted at 0.6, and the anchors are at 0 and 100, then the score is given a value of 60. Preference weights are discussed in Chap. 8—Value of health and lives.

Thresholds

Often, it is useful to define thresholds, which represent the boundaries between two categories. For example, if a threshold between high and moderate is set at 80, then a score of 83 is classified as high and a score of 77 is moderate. The way that thresholds are set is ultimately a matter of human judgement. Some people use the standard deviations of a population, others prefer round numbers.

Scales

The traditional approach is to distinguish between four scale types: nominal, ordinal, interval, and ratio [11].

Nominal

Nominal scales are simply labels, lists or classifications, with no inherent order to suggest one item is any better or worse than another. For example, parts of speech such as noun, adjective, verb, adverb etc. are nominal categories.

Ordinal

Ordinal scales allow for rank order (1st, 2nd, 3rd etc.) by which items can be sorted, such as the order of runners finishing a race. However, there is nothing to indicate the relative degree of difference between them. All that can be said is that one item is higher on the scale than another.

Interval

Interval scales are evenly spread out. Temperature in degrees Celsius is an interval scale because the difference between 10 and 20 °C is the same as the difference between 20 and 30 °C. However, it cannot be said that 20 °C is twice as hot as 10 °C. Here, 0 °C is an arbitrary anchor and we can, of course, find temperatures below 0 °C.

Ratio

In a ratio scale zero means zero. Ratio scales are used to say how many (counts) or how much (amount or magnitude) of something there is. Examples include mass, length, duration and money. The difference between two measures on an interval scale has ratio properties.

The statistical tests used for interval and ratio scales are known as parametric, while non-parametric statistics should be used for ordinal scales. Most option sets used in PROMs and PREMs have ordinal properties, but the practical differences between non-parametric and parametric tests are usually small. In this book parametric tests are used in the main, because they are more widely taught, used and understood. In every case the conclusion would be the same whether parametric or non-parametric tests were used.

Conclusions

This chapter explains some of the terms commonly used in the descriptive frameworks and scoring schemes used in PROMs and PREMs.

References

1. OECD. Skills matter: additional results from the survey of adult skills. Paris: OECD Publishing; 2019. https://doi.org/10.1787/1f029d8f-en.
2. Flesch R. A new readability yardstick. J Appl Psychol. 1948;32(3):221.
3. Gunning R. The technique of clear writing. New York: McGraw-Hill; 1952.

4. McLaughlin G. SMOG grading – a new readability formula. J Read. 1969;22:639–46.
5. Kincaid J, Fishburne R, Rogers R, Chissom B. Derivation of new readability formulas (Automatic Readability Index, Fog Count and Flesch Reading Ease Formula) for Navy enlisted personnel. US Naval Technical Training Command; 1975.
6. Lenzner T. Are readability formulas valid tools for assessing survey question difficulty? Sociol Methods Res. 2013;43(4):677–98.
7. Štajner S, Evans R, Orasan C, Mitkov R. What can readability measures really tell us about text complexity. Natural language processing for improving textual accessibility (NLP4ITA) workshop. Pompeu Fabra University, Barcelona; 2012:14–22.
8. Paz S, Jiu H, Fongwa M, et al. Readability estimates for commonly used health-related quality of life surveys. Qual Life Res. 2009;18:889–900.
9. Williamson J, Martin A. Analysis of patient information leaflets provided by a District General Hospital by the Flesch and Flesch-Kincaid method. Int J Clin Pract. 2010;64(13):1824.
10. Eremenco S, Pease S, Mann S, Berry P; PRO Consortium's Process Subcommittee. Patient-Reported Outcome (PRO) Consortium translation process: consensus development of updated best practices. J Patient Rep Outcomes. 2017;2(1):12.
11. Stevens S. On the theory of sales of measurement. Science. 1946;103:677–80.

Why PROMs Are Hard: People 4

Response Rate

Survey response rate is a good measure of success for PROMs and PREMs. We have all been asked to complete surveys. Even readers of this book, who are probably keener than most about surveys, decline far more often than they agree to take part.

The *response rate* is the proportion of people who completed a survey divided by the total number of people who should have been asked. It is useful to break this down further into two parts. Response rate is (contact rate) × (cooperation rate) where:

- *Contact rate* is the number of people asked divided by the number who should have been asked. If people are not asked to complete a survey, they will never do it.
- *Cooperation rate* is number of people who complete a survey divided by the number of people asked. Even if asked, many people will decline unless they want to do it.

Response rates have changed dramatically over time. Table 4.1 shows that response rates in 2012 were 75% down on fifteen years earlier.

Cooperation rates depend perceived relevance and burden. Few people will complete a survey they think is irrelevant, which is why the way that people are asked is vital. People need to believe that their input is going to be useful, or will benefit their own care, or that of others.

The following case study indicates some of the problems involved in obtaining good response rates in a large national survey.

Table 4.1 Response rates for telephone surveys. (*Source* Pew Research Center, 2012) [1]

	1997	2012
Contact rate (%)	90	62
Cooperation rate (%)	43	14
Response rate (%)	36	9

Case Study—GPPS

The General Practice Patient Survey (GPPS) is a large and long-running survey on patients' perceptions of GP services in England [2]. It has run since 2007 and the latest version has 61 questions with almost 3,000 words.[1]

In January 2021 the GPPS was sent to 2.4 million people. The large sample size was needed to obtain adequate samples from every general practice in England. The contact rate was high, using addresses held by the national Patient Demographic Service (PDS) database, which is kept up to date directly from GP's own computer systems.

The cooperation rate was maximized using the following methods:

1. Non responders were sent three full mailings unless they responded earlier. Each mailing included a pre-paid envelope. Each recipient was allocated a single-purpose reference number to check response. The actual survey was anonymous.
2. If a mobile telephone number was known, non-responders were also sent up to two text (SMS) reminders which included a patient-specific URL. This was added for the first time in 2021.
3. The survey could be completed in different ways (multiple modalities)—on paper, on-line or by telephone. Non-responders were identified after allowing for opt outs, deaths and other reasons.
4. The survey could be completed in English and in 14 other languages—2.5% of responses were in languages other than English.
5. Every GP surgery was provided with posters for their waiting rooms.
6. Telephone helplines were provided.
7. The text was tested in advance and checked for clarity by the Campaign for Plain English.
8. The invitation letter was worded to emphasize local as well as national benefits.
9. All results, including those for every general practice, were published on a dedicated web-site (https://gp-patient.co.uk/).

---

[1] GPPS covers: local GP services (8 questions), making an appointment (12 questions), last appointment (9 questions), overall experience (1 question), own health (10 questions), when GP practice is closed (4 questions), NHS dentistry (4 questions), COVID-19 (2 questions), and demographic details (11 questions).

10. Most questions (75%) were kept the same year-to-year enabling data trends to be seen. Fifteen changes were introduced in 2021 because of changes in priorities, legislation and COVID.
11. Full technical details have been published ensuring transparency (https://www.gp-patient.co.uk/Downloads/2021/GPPS_2021_Technical_Annex_PUBLIC.pdf).
12. A set of case studies have been published showing how the survey has been used nationally, regionally, locally and for academic research.

It is hard to imagine what more might be done, other than making it shorter. Even so, the response rate fell from 44% in 2007 to 31% in 2020, before increasing to almost 35% in 2021. It is too early to know whether the rise in 2021 was due to improved communication efforts, increased on-line completion (up from 6% in 2017 to 37% in 2021), COVID-19 lockdown or a combination of these.

Issues that work in the opposite direction include:

1. The survey is long (61 questions and 2,984 words). The invitation letter was also long with 861 words (total 3845 words).
2. The reading age requirements are fairly high. For the survey, the Flesch Kincaid Grade (FKG) is 6.1 (reading age 11–12) and, for the first invitation letter, the FKG is 8.1 (reading age 13–14).
3. According to the invitation letter, the survey takes 15 min to complete. The Technical Annex estimates that respondents devoted 173,115 hours to completing the survey.
4. Results were not published until six months after the survey was sent out.
5. People cannot see how their own response compares with others, locally or nationally.
6. For people under 35 the response rate was under 20%. This rose to over 65% for those aged 65 to 85. Older people make more use of NHS services.
7. Response rate for women (39.9%) was higher than for men (30.8%). This may be because women take on more responsibility for their family's health care.
8. Response rate was lower in deprived areas, which have more people with ethnic minority backgrounds, single, separated, divorced and unemployed people, and households with three or more people or privately rented. In 7% of practices the response rate was below 20%, while in 16% of practices it was over 50%.

This case study shows some of the barriers to obtaining high response rates and how these can be ameliorated. People often ask, 'what's in it for me?' before deciding whether to cooperate. A long survey is always a barrier. For comparison, the GPPS (excluding invitation letter) is two-thirds the length of this chapter.

Digital Exclusion

Digital exclusion is about not having the access, skills, and confidence to use the internet and so digitally excluded people cannot benefit from using digital technology in everyday life [3]. The COVID-19 pandemic has encouraged more people to go online, but in 2021 about 5% of the UK population remain digitally excluded and a further 24% do not use the digital devices for email, health care or banking [4].

Lack of access is related to connectivity issues, affordability and need for assistive technology. Using the internet needs basic digital capability for day-to-day tasks. Confidence is related to trust in the technology and in oneself to do things right and avoid risks such as scams. People need the motivation to see why the Internet is relevant and useful for them.

Younger people (digital natives) have been brought up with the Internet, Wi-Fi, smart-phones, and tablets; they find it hard to imagine how people lived without them. For older people, these are new innovations. They have adopted them according to their level of innovativeness (see below). Many people do not have the right technology at home (e.g., Wi-Fi), nor appropriate skills. Many patients are old, infirm or have cognitive challenges such as dementia [5].

Globally, internet access is still increasing at about 7% per annum. By 2021, more than 60% of the global population was connected to the Internet. In Northern Europe this was 97%, followed by Western Europe at 93%. About 90% of internet users use a smartphone, and almost 70% also say they use a laptop or desktop computer to access the internet. The gap is smallest in Western Europe. Older people are more likely to use computers and tablets than mobiles [6].

Innovation Readiness

The concept of innovation readiness, or innovativeness, is based on Everett Rogers' classic text on innovation diffusion [7]. Rogers originally developed these ideas by studying the adoption of new farming practices in Iowa during the 1950s but soon recognized that these concepts are universal.

Diffusion and dissemination of innovation are complementary concepts. The term *spread* covers both diffusion and dissemination.

- Diffusion is horizontal, usually unplanned and subjective, through informal peer networks.
- Dissemination is vertical, planned, and targeted top-down from the center. It is often based on experts' recommendations.

In healthcare we find both diffusion and dissemination. Spread happens most rapidly when these two forces work together. A good example is the way that home working and video conferencing developed during the COVID-19 pandemic.

The introduction of anything new, including PROMs or PREMs, should be thought of as an innovation needing spread.

Innovativeness Spectrum

Innovativeness is the degree to which an individual or organization is relatively earlier or later in adopting new ideas than other members of the system. At the individual level, members of a social system may be classified into adopter categories based on innovativeness. The main groups are innovators, early adopters, early majority (pragmatists), late majority (conservatives), and laggards. These groups differ a lot between groups and in how much value they put on any specific innovation.

Innovators

Typically, innovators are often technology enthusiasts, geeks or pioneers. They recognize the potential of an innovation, even if it does not work quite as it should. They will spend hours of their own time helping to make it better.

Innovators are rare, comprising between 0 and 2.5% of any target market. Assuming a normal distribution, innovators are more than two standard deviations above average. In IQ terms, they are as easy to find as people in the general population with an IQ of more than 130.

Early Adopters

Early adopters are key to the success of any innovation. They are visionaries who can see how a new technology can match a strategic opportunity. Early adopters tend to be optimistic, open, and well informed about new ideas. They have the temperament to make an innovation work and the ability to sell it within their organization. They also tend to be demanding, capable and respected locally. They may take calculated risks but recognize that they are at the leading (bleeding) edge. If it does not work out, they rapidly move on.

Early adopters are more common than innovators but still rare. They represent about 13.5% of the target market. In statistical terms they are between one and two standard deviations more innovative than average. In IQ terms they are as common as people in the population with an IQ between 115 and 130.

Often, a successful innovation is launched by an innovator working with an early adopter to make it happen.

Early Majority

The early majority are pragmatists, who deliberate carefully before choosing. They comprise about one third of the target market.

There is a big difference between early adopters and the early majority. The early majority are risk-averse; they expect things to work perfectly from the start and they value quality, service, and reliability. Having chosen a course, they tend to be loyal.

For any business, changing focus from early adopters to the early majority is hard. Large numbers fail at this stage. It is described as crossing the chasm [8].

The early majority are up to one standard deviation faster than the mean and represent about one third of the target market. They are mainstream customers for any successful innovation.

Late Majority

The late majority are conservative. They are skeptical of change. However, they make up a third of the target market—there are lots of them. The late majority are up to one standard deviation slower than average to adopt a new idea.

It is a mistake to ignore the late majority because they can be very effective at blocking innovations they dislike. The late majority tend to be older and in senior positions. Many businesses make a good living from selling mature innovations to the late majority, treating them as cash cows.

Laggards

Laggards are traditionalists; they don't like any change. These are slower than one standard deviation below the mean.

In practice, many laggards never adopt an innovation before they retire. The tail of the innovation cycle can be spread out over decades until the last laggard retires, dies or is left with no other option.

Individual people (patients and staff) differ greatly, as indicated by the broad spectrum of innovativeness. Each innovativeness category has characteristic differences in terms of personality values, communication behavior, demographics and capability of getting what they want.

Decision Process

The innovation-decision process is the process of understanding the advantages and disadvantages of doing or using something. It starts once a need has been expressed or recognized and includes the following general steps, which may or may not be explicit:

- Knowledge acquisition
- Persuade
- Decide (adopt or reject)
- Implement
- Confirm, evaluate and promote.

The rate of adoption is measured by how long it takes for a certain proportion of the members of a system to use the innovation. Innovators and early adopters have much shorter decision periods than late adopters and laggards.

Aspects of innovations, such as PROMs and PREMs, that help explain different adoption rates include its relative advantage (is it better than what it replaces?), compatibility, complexity, trialability, observability or visibility, adaptability and the evidence base.

Within organizations, the innovation-decision process may be more structured:

- Agenda—identify a need
- Match—fit a solution to the problem
- Redefine/restructure—adapt the organization and/or the innovation to each other
- Clarify—the meaning of the innovation becomes clearer to the organization's members
- Routinise—the innovation is widely used and sustainable. It is the way we do things here.

Innovation almost always involves adaptive change, which puts pressure on staff at all levels. Attributes for success include a culture of receptiveness to new ideas and the organization's capability, capacity, and perseverance to make new ideas work.

These processes apply to all types of change, including the PROMs and PREMs lifecycle.

Change Management

A lesson from all health innovation studies (including PROMs and PREMs) is that change takes time and needs effort, capability, capacity, and perseverance. If you try to implement something that is not fit for purpose you will inevitably fail, but good solutions have no guarantees of success either. Understanding the social dimension and having the right culture and approach are critical.

Progress often comes from small incremental changes, which accumulate to deliver large gains over the medium term. Successful change is driven by a combination of technical, policy, economic, clinical or managerial factors working together on different actors and at different levels within organizations [9].

Common factors include:

- Technology developments, such as Wi-Fi and mobile technologies.
- Culture of clinicians and managers working well together.
- Detailed re-design of patient-centered pathways to give better outcomes at lower cost.
- Data sharing, plus appropriate performance metrics that enable feedback, benchmarking and comparisons of performance and variation.
- Frontline support, such as quality improvement, education and training and dissemination of best practice.
- Financial carrots and sticks that incentivize and focus attention on the need for change.

Table 4.2 Errors and remedies in management of change

Common errors	Proposed remedy
1. Not establish a great enough sense of urgency	Establish a sense of urgency that something really has to be done (it may help to have a crisis)
2. Fail to create a sufficiently powerful guiding coalition	Form a powerful guiding coalition of key stakeholders with position power, expertise, credibility and leadership
3. Underestimate the power of vision	Create a vision and strategy that is desirable, feasible, focused, flexible and can be communicated in less than five minutes
4. Under-communicate the vision by a factor of 10 or more	Communicate the change vision simply using examples. This needs to be repeated over again in multiple forums; address apparent inconsistencies, listen and be listened to
5. Permit obstacles to block the new vision	Empower employees to modify structures and systems to bring about the changes required. Almost certainly, changes will be needed in process, workflow and information systems
6. Fail to create short-term wins	Generate short-term wins that are visible, clearly related to the change effort and build momentum
7. Declare victory too soon	Consolidate gains, reduce interdependencies and create more change
8. Neglect to anchor changes firmly in the corporate culture	Anchor new approaches in the culture. This comes last, not first

Kotter identifies eight common errors and proposes remedies for managing innovation and change (Table 4.2) [10].

In this section we also discuss three important techniques which are important in any innovation or change management project: behavior change, the Plan-Do-Study-Act (PDSA) cycle and SMART criteria.

Behavior Change

Many projects start with a chief executive or politician wanting to make a change top-down from the center. However, change requires people to change their behavior, so we need to think bottom-up about why and how people change their behavior. Introducing PROMs and PREMs is an innovative change.

Michie's Behavior Change Wheel (BCW) helps us understand how we can successfully introduce changes in behavior and culture at the level of individuals, communities, and populations [11]. It incorporates two valuable ideas: the COM-B model of behavior change, and behavior change techniques (BCT).

According to US criminal law, to prove someone is guilty of a crime you have to demonstrate the means or capability, opportunity and motive. Motivation, Opportunity and Capability, along with Behavior itself, are the components of the COM-B Model.

The *sine qua non* of PROMs and PREMs is that people complete the surveys, and we obtain a good response rate.

Capability

People need the capability to do it. This includes both the psychological and physical capacity to engage in an activity, including the necessary knowledge, skills, and tools. If people cannot complete a survey, we need to arrange for an adequate proxy to do it on their behalf. For small children, a parent is usually used; for people with dementia or the frail elderly, a caregiver or family member may be suitable. Sometimes we have to fall back on a member of staff.

Opportunity

People also need the opportunity for the behavior to occur. Opportunity includes everything that makes a behavior possible or prompts it. Opportunity has social and physical aspects. If you carry a tablet, you have the physical opportunity to use it, although this may not be socially acceptable at a dinner party. For surveys, only ask people to complete the survey when and where they have full access to any technology required.

Motivation

People need motivation. They must be more highly motivated to do what we want (complete a survey) than to do something else. Motivation includes both unconscious habits and conscious thoughts and goals. These relate to fast automatic thinking (System 1) and slow reflective thinking (System 2), which work in very different ways [12]. If people think that doing what is asked is easy and beneficial, then they will do it. If not, they won't [13]. This is a reason why respondent burden is critical.

Capability and Opportunity also influence Motivation.

Behavior Change

Behavior change is what we seek or try to understand. Capability, Opportunity and Motivation each influence Behavior and are influenced by Behavior in turn. To alter Behavior, you need to be clear about what you want to happen (e.g., complete a survey) and the context in which that can be achieved. Then think about what is needed to achieve that. For one type of behavior change it may be most appropriate to remove a barrier by improving some aspect of Capability, while for another it may be best to deter by restricting the Opportunity to do something else.

Many different *behavioral change techniques* (BCTs) have been identified [14]. These include setting goals and planning, feedback and monitoring, social support, shaping knowledge, natural consequences, comparison of behavior, associations, repetition and substitution, comparison of outcomes, reward and threat, regulation, antecedents, identity, scheduled consequences, self-belief, and covert learning. One of the skills is knowing when to use each one.

We discuss planning using the PDSA cycle.

PDSA Cycle

The PDSA (Plan-Do-Study-Act) cycle is a cornerstone of quality improvement. It was originally introduced by Shewhart in the 1920s and later popularized and improved by Deming [15].

Plan

We must be crystal clear about what we are trying to achieve and how we recognize success. This may involve interim steps such as identifying the changes needed.

It is useful to make predictions about what we expect to happen and to measure whether these are being achieved using SMART measures (see below). You can't improve what you do not measure.

There is no point in asking any question if everyone already knows the answer. The interesting questions are those where the answer is not obvious, or where people disagree about predictions. Often our best guess about what will happen turns out wrong. This is how we find out new things, so it is important that the questions we ask help us understand what is really going on.

This stage is also when we set out our plans about how to collect the data required—what questions are to be asked, by whom, when, where and how. This is the foundation on which everything else builds, so effort at the Plan stage is always worthwhile.

Do

This is the data collection stage. If the Plan is good, then Do may be relatively simple, but all the people involved must know exactly what is expected of them.

Study

Study is the analysis of the data to identify changes and trends over time and to present the results in a way that is easily understood by those who need to use them. Results should be compared to predictions or previous results.

Act

This is acting on the results, planning the next change cycle or spreading implementation further.

PDSA cycles can run sequentially or even simultaneously. If they run simultaneously, in parallel, it is useful to ensure that the outcomes and questions used are coordinated, because a change in one area can impact others.

It is safer to start on a small scale, to capture what you learn, adapt the methods and then increase the numbers in a planned way. Also test ideas first with people who believe in what you are trying to achieve. It is never easy to convert sceptics without any evidence.

SMART Criteria

Ideally objectives should be quantified. It is easier to compare numbers than qualitative judgements and impressions. SMART (Specific, Measurable, Assignable, Realistic and Time-bound) criteria are used widely in quality improvement work for setting goals and objectives [16]. They can be applied to PROMs and PREMs projects.

Specific

Objectives should identify a specific area for improvement. There may be multiple objectives but each one should be specified in terms of the result desired. Instead of saying *achieve better patient well-being*, which is not specific, the objective should be *improve average patient wellbeing by 10 points using the Patient Well-being Score*. Sometimes scores are already high, so in these cases it may be important to add a supplementary objective such as *or be above 90*. Ensure that specific objectives do not create perverse incentives.

Measurable

Each objective should be measurable, using a pre-defined quantitative metric. It should be clear what is a good or a bad result, so people know whether they have met the objective or not. Measurable objectives are motivating. One reason to use PROMs and PREMs is to provide numbers (quantitative data), not just qualitative anecdotes.

Assignable

Objectives must be assigned to the right person. Each objective should be achievable because of the efforts of the person, or team, to whom it is assigned. That person or team must own the objective.

Realistic

Objectives should be challenging but not so challenging that there is little chance of success given available resources. They need to be achieved using the tools that each person has available and recognize factors that are outside their control.

For example, it is not realistic to expect all patients to score 100 on the Personal Wellbeing Score. An improvement of 10 points may well be achievable, but this depends on case-mix and other factors.

Time-Bound

SMART objectives state the time when each objective will be achieved. For example, the time scale for personal wellbeing may be the interval between two events, such as between first appointment and follow-up two months later, or year-on-year. It may be easier to improve patient well-being before and after an episode of care than at annual follow-ups.

Conclusions

This chapter has covered some of the problems of introducing PROMs and PREMs, involving people and organizations, and what can be done to overcome these.

The innovation spectrum and change management techniques, including PDSA and SMART, are discussed.

The next chapter deals with the problems of noise, bias and complexity, which are inevitable in this domain.

References

1. Kohut A, Keeter S, Doherty C, et al. Assessing the representativeness of public opinion surveys. Washington DC: Pew Research Centre; 2012.
2. GP Patient Survey 2021: Technical Annexe. London, Ipsos MORI 2021 (https://www.gp-patient.co.uk/Downloads/2021/GPPS_2021_Technical_Annex_PUBLIC.pdf. Accessed 13 July 2021.
3. Stone E. Digital exclusion and health inequalities: briefing paper. London: Good Things Foundation; 2021.
4. Lloyds Bank UK. Consumer digital index, 6th edn. Lloyds; 2021.
5. Kontos E, Blake KD, Chou W-YS, et al. Predictors of e-health usage: insights on the digital divide from the health information national trends survey 2012. J Med Internet Res. 2014;16: e172.
6. Global Web Index. London: GWI; 2021.
7. Rogers E. Diffusion of innovations. 5th ed. New York NY: Free Press; 2003.
8. Moore G. Crossing the chasm: harnessing and selling disruptive products to mainstream customers, 3rd edn. New York, NY: Harper Collins; 2014.
9. Alderwick H, Roberton R, Appleby J, Dunn P, Maguire D. Better value in the NHS: the role of changes in clinical practice. London: The Kings Fund; 2015.
10. Kotter J. Leading change. Harvard Business School Press; 1996.
11. Michie S, van Stralen M, West R. The behaviour change wheel: a new method for characterising and designing behaviour change interventions. Implement Sci. 2011;6:42.
12. Kahneman D. Thinking, fast and slow. Penguin; 2012.
13. Thaler R, Sunstein C. Nudge: the final edition. Penguin; 2021.
14. Michie S, Richardson M, Johnston M, et al. The behavior change technique taxonomy (v1) of 93 hierarchically clustered techniques: building an international consensus for the reporting of behavior change interventions. Ann Behav Med. 2013;46(1):81–95.
15. Deming WE. Out of the crisis. Boston: MIT CAES; 1982.
16. Doran G. There's a SMART way to write management's goals and objectives. Manag Rev. 1981;70(11):35–6.

Noise and Complexity

Noise and Bias

Answering any survey question always involves the following four steps of understanding the question, retrieving relevant information from memory, deciding which response option fits best, and responding in a way that fits the judgement.

Raters may try to save effort by doing one or more of these steps sub-optimally creating noise and bias. Risks increase if surveys are answered in private without another person present to sense-check responses, if the survey is long or difficult, it is seen as a chore, or it is not regarded as relevant [1].

Noise and bias are related error types.

Noise is unwanted variability in judgments (scatter) where you would expect people to make the same decisions from the same information. Examples include diagnosis and treatment decisions. Noise matters because it leads to errors, unfairness and inconsistent decision-making. Even if judgements are correct on average, noise judgement errors do not cancel out.

Bias occurs when most errors in a set of judgments are offset in the same direction.

PROMs and PREMs ask respondents about their perceptions or judgments. Judgment is a form of measurement in which the instrument is the human mind. Like other measurements, a judgment assigns a score, usually a number. It helps to think of this score as a number with an error component.

Much of this section is based on *Noise: a flaw in human judgment* by Kahneman, Sibony and Sunstein, which is recommended reading [2].

The error in a single measurement is bias plus noisy error, where bias is the average error of all measurements and noisy error is the residual error or scatter of each measure. Noise averages out to zero across all measurements.

The standard way to measure accuracy is the mean squared error (MSE), which is $(bias)^2 + (noise)^2$. MSE is always positive and treats positive and negative errors the same. Using MSE, noise and bias are independent and additive sources of error.

The squaring of bias and noise indicates the importance of avoiding both large amounts of either bias or noise.

Our goal is always to minimise noise and bias. These have equal weighting, but noise is often the bigger problem. If judgments are normally distributed, the effect of noise and bias are equal when 84% of judgments are biased (higher or lower than the mean). If bias is smaller than one standard deviation, then noise is the bigger source of error. This is usually the case.

Types of Noise

There are three main types of noise: level noise, stable pattern noise and occasion noise.

Level Noise

Level noise is the variability or scatter of average judgments made by different people, who might be expected to agree with each other. Level noise is often due to the questionnaire itself. Human language is ambiguous. Different people understand questions and options in different ways, based more on differences in their understanding of each question than on any real difference between people. Therefore, survey designers have a responsibility to check that all people understand the language and terms used in the same way.

Stable Pattern Noise

Stable pattern noise reflects the respondents. Some people are optimists, and others are pessimists. Some will always mark high, and others always mark low. When using long option scales, some people will always avoid the extremities, while others do not. Long option scales are often the largest source of noise.

Occasion Noise

Occasion noise is transient variation. Some people will tend to score lower in the afternoon than in the morning, if they are hungry or if their favourite football team has just lost. To minimise occasion noise, it is good practice to ask people how they felt yesterday or in the past 24 hours, rather than right now.

Types of Bias

Bias has been studied extensively but is only a problem if we are trying to make accurate predictions, such as who will win an election. In many studies involving PROMs and PREMs we compare two measures, such as before and after or one month with another. If both are equally biased, the difference is accurate. However this is not true of noise. If two people give different judgments about the same thing (e.g., making a diagnosis), at least one of them is always wrong.

Bias falls into several broad categories: cognitive bias, statistical bias and contextual bias. Wikipedia lists more than 45 different types of bias [3]. Some of these are discussed below.

Cognitive Bias

Cognitive biases include: anchoring based on an initial frame of reference, confirmation bias, the halo effect, patternicity, which is seeing a pattern in random events, cultural bias and framing, self-serving bias, when people give answers that are in their own best interests, and status quo bias that favours the current state of affairs.

Several cognitive biases are found in surveys. People are often unwilling to criticise harshly those who care for them (self-serving bias). If they answered the first question positively, they are more likely to answer other questions in the same way (anchoring). They are also less likely to answer questions in a way that is contrary to social norms or their own beliefs (cultural and confirmation bias).

Statistical Bias

Statistical bias is any issue in data collection that leads to lopsided results. This can be caused by sample selection. For example, when surveys are used to predict results in election polls, the wrong answer may result if one part of the population was not asked the survey or decided not to vote.

Forecast bias is found when people consistently forecast high or low. This can be an issue in medicine, where many diseases are self-limiting. People attribute a cure for a medical intervention in conditions that would get better naturally without treatment.

For example, when I was a child, tonsillectomy (surgical removal of tonsils) was performed frequently and caused many deaths. It is now rare because most children get better without surgery. I was lucky to survive a post-tonsillectomy haemorrhage, many did not.

The observer effect is when the researcher unconsciously biases the results—in clinical trials this is a reason for using double-blind studies.

Selection bias refers to the way that groups are selected. Much psychology research has been criticised as being largely based on WEIRD samples. WEIRD is an acronym for Western, Educated, Industrialised, Rich and Democratic [4].

Contextual Bias

Contextual and cultural bias include: reporting bias—publishing results that agree with the original hypothesis—health inequalities, such as the inverse care law and many types of prejudice such as sexism, ageism and racialism. Contextual bias is found in academia, law enforcement, media, education, commerce, health care, sport and gambling.

Reducing Noise and Bias

Kahneman, Sibony and Sunstein propose six principles of decision hygiene, which apply to reducing both noise and bias [2].

The goal is accuracy, not individual expression

People are inconsistent at distinguishing between similar things. One way of avoiding this is to ensure that questions are quick and easy to answer, are unambiguous and limit the opportunity for individuality. Short option scales (e.g. 4 options) are better than long scales (e.g. 11 options) in helping people rate similar things the same way.

Think statistically, and take an outside view of the case

It is always helpful to word surveys in ways that help people be consistent with how others would rate the same thing. An example is to use words taught in primary schools. This aids predictions.

Structure judgments into several independent tasks

People are often inconsistent in how they weight multiple dimensions of an issue. If people say A is similar to B it does not mean that they mean B is similar to A. For example, people may agree that Oxford is like London but disagree that London is like Oxford. This is a universal property of human beings. It is one reason why multi-attribute utility estimation is so hard. In health state preference judgments, people are inconsistent when asked to trade off quality of life against length of life (see Chap. 8).

Avoid asking the same question in different ways, unless this is what you set out to do, such as in school tests. For each issue it is best to make a list of each critical component, ensuring that each is largely independent of the others, and ask about these one at a time.

Resist premature intuitions

Good decision hygiene is to answer each attribute-specific question before making a global evaluation. Confirmation bias is the tendency of people to notice, believe and recall information that confirms what they said earlier. To avoid this, it is better to go from the specific to the general, not the other way round. For example, ask about pain, anxiety and disability separately before asking about overall health. This avoids leaving out information that may turn out to be important overall.

Obtain independent judgments from multiple judges, then consider aggregating those judgments

Judgments from multiple independent people are better than those from one person only. However, the judges must be fully independent. Keep people apart until you need a consensus. Surveys do this naturally.

Favour relative judgments and relative scales

People find it easier to perform pairwise comparisons than most other forms of judgment. For example, a four-point scale of Strongly agree, Agree, Disagree, Strongly disagree can be broken down into two simple comparisons. First: agree or disagree. Second, if agree: strongly agree or agree; or if disagree: strongly disagree or disagree. Respondents find this easier than allocating a numerical score directly.

These principles are based on modern behavioural psychology research. All are important. Key aspects are summarised in Fig. 5.1. They underpin most of the recommendations about survey design and judgments made throughout this book.

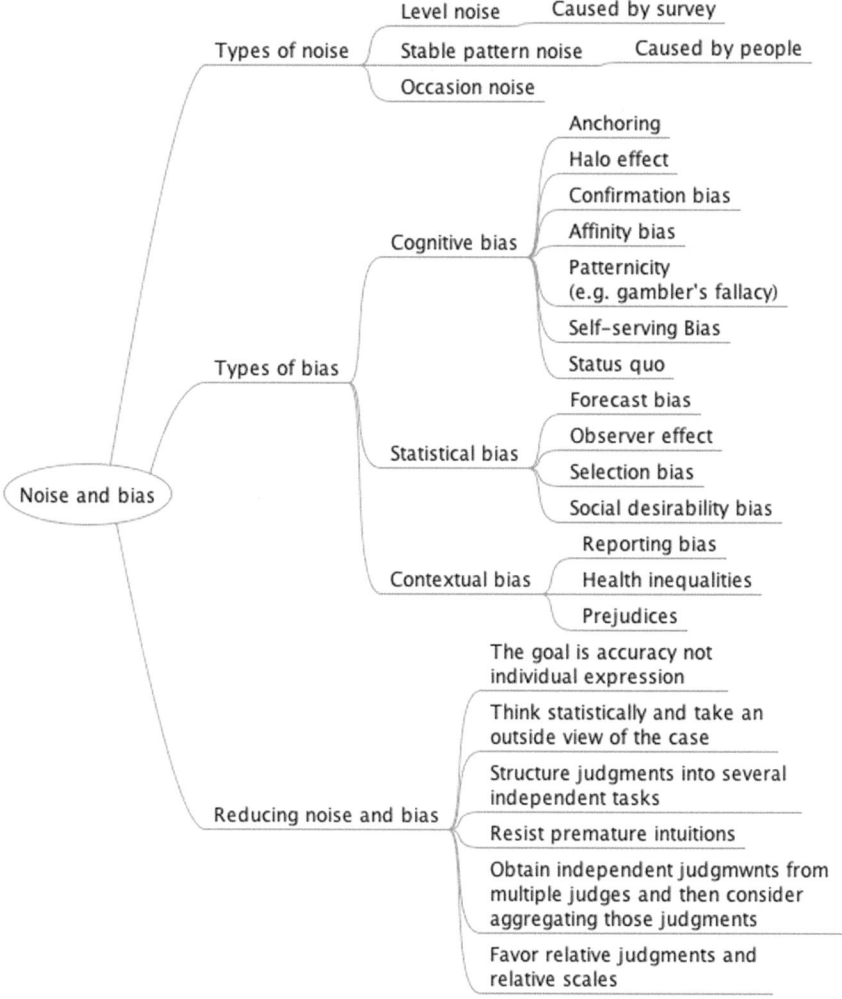

Fig. 5.1 Types of noise and bias

Complexity

Complexity Theory

Complexity is inescapable when working in healthcare. In complexity theory, systems can be simple, complicated or complex.

Simple systems have a cause-and-effect relationship, which is easy to understand.

Complicated systems are harder to understand but still follow the cause-and-effect pathway. Complicated systems usually have multiple components and, if everything works correctly, always produce the desired result. Examples include large computer programs.

Complex problems are different because they are intrinsically unpredictable. Healthcare is usually described as a complex adaptive system, which has many dynamically interacting parts. Each part of the system is affected by and affects several other parts. Interactions can be non-linear, and small changes may have large effects.

A well-known example of complexity is deterministic chaos. Here, the exact present state, exactly determines the future, but oddly the approximate present does not approximately represent the future. Tiny differences in initial conditions, such as those due to rounding numbers, can lead to widely diverging outcomes, rendering long-term prediction impossible. A famous illustration is the *Butterfly Effect*, which is the idea that a butterfly flapping its wings in Brazil may set off a tornado in Texas [5]. Another example is a double pendulum—a pendulum with another pendulum attached to its end. The path of the end of the second pendulum is sensitive to minute changes in the initial conditions.

No system is more complex or as hard to change as healthcare [6]. The system boundaries are vague. Present behaviour is shaped by the past, but some parts are unaware of the behaviour of big picture and respond mainly to is in front of them.

Two examples of well-intentioned change projects in England, which turned into disasters, were:

- The National Programme for Information Technology (NPfIT), launched in 2002, was intended to transform healthcare [7]. In reality, it did far more harm than good. It cost over £13 billion ($20 billion) before being abandoned. It achieved very few of its objectives and decimated the UK healthcare computing industry.
- The Lansley reorganisation of the NHS, which was launched in 2010, was intended to increase competition between health care providers [8]. It has been reversed because integration (joined-up care) is more important than competition. Integration requires collaboration, while competition favours winner takes all.

On the other hand, there are plenty of examples of how the health care systems have responded positively. These include:

- Adoption of new diagnostic tests and imaging technology, medicines and surgical advances, such as laparoscopic surgery.
- Vaccination and other public health measures.
- Remote consultations and other responses to the COVID pandemic.

Braithwaite suggests six principles to guide healthcare quality improvement [9]:

1. Focus on how care is delivered at the coalface.
2. Meaningful improvement is local and centred on natural networks of clinicians and patients.
3. Clinicians get things right far more often than not. Use clinicians to help identify the factors and conditions that underpin success.
4. Common success factors include starting small, being open and transparent, being collaborative and putting the patient at the centre.
5. Recognise that change is hard won, takes time and needs to be adapted to its setting. Change usually requires substantial local support to make it work well.
6. We don't know in advance how it will work out.

NASSS Framework

Greenhalgh's NASSS framework helps us understand the reasons for failure of complex digital innovations, in terms of Non-adoption, Abandonment and failure to Scale, Sustain or Spread [10]. People who want to find out more are encouraged to read the original paper.

The NASSS framework (see Fig. 5.2) decomposes the healthcare system in seven levels, summarised below. A problem at just one of level is often enough to derail the roll out of a technology that has been shown to be successful elsewhere. Issues at multiple levels are a recipe for failure.

Condition

Health care is organized around different groups of diseases and treatments, but the natural histories of different diseases vary enormously. The International Classification of Diseases (ICD-11) contains 55,000 types of disease, injury and cause of death.

A single condition can have a lot of variation. The COVID pandemic demonstrates how hard it is to deal with just one disease. Outcomes range from complete recovery through chronic disease (long COVID), acute care and death. Different outcome measures may be appropriate at each stage in the natural history of the disease. Severely ill people may not be able answer survey questions themselves.

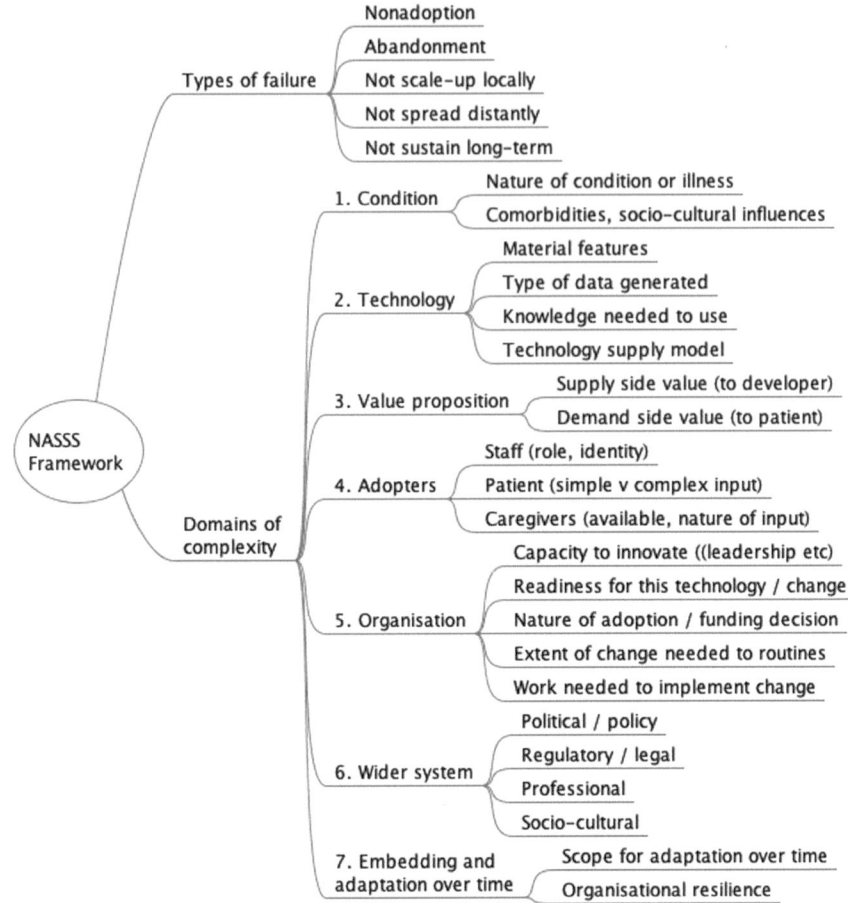

Fig. 5.2 NASSS Framework, (based on Greenhalgh et al. [10])

Thousands of condition-specific PROMs have been developed, mainly for use in drug clinical trials. Trial results are used to support applications to regulators, such as the FDA. These studies usually exclude people with multiple conditions, which creates two problems. First, drugs are frequently given to people with disease combinations that have not been evaluated. Second, the PROMs used in clinical trials were not usually designed for people living with more than one condition.

Most money in health care is spent on people living with multiple conditions. The number of possible combinations is vast. A good treatment for one condition can aggravate another.

An alternative approach is to use generic PROMs. The term generic applies to outcome and experience measures that are not specific to any particular specialty, condition, mode of treatment or other population sub-group. Most of the measures described in this book are generic.

Technology

All aspects of the technology used must work satisfactorily.

Technology evolves all the time, which creates its own problems. What is in place already may determine whether new technologies can be easily adopted and adapted to meet local constraints. It also affects patients' perception of benefits, depending on the starting point.

Survey results must invariably be processed through a computer, but this may create problems if the respondents are not digitally literate. Digital literacy covers not only the skills needed to use systems, but also those needed to sort out any difficulties or errors if there is no one available to help. Systems need to be easy to use and reliable.

The people who are least likely to be digitally literate are those in their last couple of years of life, when most healthcare expenditure is incurred. These patients often find themselves on the wrong side of the digital divide and may live alone.

Many patients find tablets, such as iPads linked to WiFi, easier to use for data collection than either personal computers or smartphones. Tablets are readily portable to where the patient is, require little manual dexterity, and can and be used for surveys or video.

Clinicians use a wide range of different computer systems, such as electronic patient records (EPR) or specialised clinical systems, but EPR systems seldom process PROMs or PREMs well.

Technology rapidly becomes out of date, so there is always a problem of older systems migrating to or coexisting alongside newer ones. Systems can be vulnerable to obsolescence, supplier withdrawal or take-over.

Computers use codes, but standard coding schemes, such as SNOMED CT, do not contain the codes needed for PROMs and PREMs (see Chap. 7). This has led suppliers to develop their own codes and terms, which do not interoperate.

Healthcare interoperability is widely recognised to be a major problem [11]. In part this is a direct consequence of the technology supply model and competition, as companies attempt to retain their existing market through customer and data lock-in (see Chap. 7).

Value Proposition

The value proposition set out by different stakeholders to sell their offerings is inevitably targeted at their audience. Suppliers need to sell their wares to potential purchasers; managers need to sell changes to their staff. The success of each value proposition depends on how people receive it. This depends on the persuasiveness of the arguments used and the arguments used depend on the audience.

The value propositions set out by different actors may not be the same. Salesmen have every incentive to magnify benefits and minimise problems. The value to the developer is related to expected return on investment. If this is based on unrealistic sales assumptions, the business may not survive.

The value to the purchaser, clinician and patient depends on accurate assessment that the proposed system is affordable, desirable, safe and effective. Affordability is often paramount. For most healthcare providers, being more effective (better outcomes and experience) does not generate more short-term revenue.

As outlined in Chap. 4, many innovations fail to cross the chasm between early adopters and the early majority. These two groups see the value proposition in different ways. Early adopters are visionary and will accept risk, but the early majority is pragmatic and dislikes risk.

Adopters (Staff, Patients and Caregivers)

Individual patients, healthcare professionals and managers vary enormously in their willingness to embrace change, from innovators and early adopters through to late majority and laggards (see Chap. 4) [12].

The Association of American Medical Colleges (AAMC) recognizes 135 specialties and subspecialties. In the UK the General Medical Council (GMC) approves the curricula and assessments of 65 specialties and 31 sub-specialties. The proliferation of medical specialties is driven by specialization and division of labour, leading to multiple silos. For many doctors, their income and reputation depends at least as much on recognition within their specialty, nationally and internationally than locally within their healthcare provider. People in each specialty speak their own dialect of medicine.

Some staff simply do not wish to engage in using PROMs and PREMs. Some reasons are due to technology issues (see above) but more commonly there is perceived self-interest involved. Some see PROMs as making more work. This includes the time needed to ask the questions and review the results, to learn new skills or to deal with issues that had remained hidden previously. Others fear a threat to their own autonomy and self-confidence. Many are content with the way that they have always done things. The consequence of not engaging is seldom severe.

Organizations

Every healthcare organization has its own local culture, capabilities and resources, which constrains what can be done. Peter Drucker is quoted as saying: *culture eats strategy for breakfast*. Culture change is hard.

Organizations are usually reluctant to innovate if they have weak leadership, staff shortages, little money and are risk averse. Sometimes opponents with vested interests can wreck a sound plan. Change is always easier when there is adequate funding, tension for change, wide support, few barriers to overcome and a willingness to take calculated risks.

Organizations often reject change if the primary strategy is to mandate solutions from the top down and the initiative encounters entrenched bureaucracy or conflicts with existing policies and procedures. Work is always needed to build a shared vision, engage staff, enact new ways of working and monitor impact. The shared vision needs to be clear about what the technology can and cannot do.

Wider Context

Governments, regulators and professional bodies can promote, enable or inhibit changes in ways that are hard to predict. These aspects include health policy (including care models), fiscal policy (including funding), professional and regulatory body positions and legal and regulatory issues. For example, information governance regulations are mainly set by governments. It is not a good omen if proposed changes are actively opposed by parties with the power to mobilise, resist or reject, such as the medical trade unions or the media.

Embedding and Adaption Over Time

These levels are interlinked and evolve over time in ways that are unpredictable. Systems and people need time to make new ideas their own. The system must be sufficiently flexible to respond to changed circumstances, but how this is best done cannot be prescribed in advance. For example, no one before 2020 predicted the impact of the COVID pandemic, nor how health services would respond. There are many other examples of the impact of unpredicted events. Successful innovations can be adapted to new circumstances.

NASSS provides a useful checklist to ensure that all bases are covered. Some tools used to measure the digital readiness of people and organisations are described in Chap. 16 on innovation evaluation.

Conclusions

Chapters 4 and 5 provides a list of many difficulties involved with introducing PROMs and PREMs (and other innovations) into health care settings. They help explain why progress has been slow. These ideas have been explored elsewhere, but not in the context of PROMs and PREMs. However, things do change, and innovation does happen, so all these obstacles can be avoided or overcome. It is always easier if barriers are recognised in advance and avoided whenever possible.

References

1. Krosnick JA. Response strategies for coping with the cognitive demands of attitude measures in surveys. Appl Cogn Psychol. 1991;5(3):213–36.
2. Kahneman D, Sibony O, Sunstein CS. Noise—a flaw in human judgment. London: Collins; 2021.
3. https://en.wikipedia.org/wiki/Bias. Accessed 20 October 2021.
4. Henrich J, Heine SJ, Norenzayan A. The weirdest people in the world? Behav Brain Sci. 2010;33:61–83.
5. Gleick J. Chaos: making a new science. Cardinal Books; 1987.
6. May C, Cummings A, Girling M, et al. Using normalization process theory in feasibility studies and process evaluations of complex healthcare interventions: a systematic review. Implement Sci. 2018;13(1):1–27.

7. Wachter R. Making IT work: harnessing the power of health information technology to improve care in England. London, UK: Department of Health; 2016.
8. Timmins N. The World's biggest quango: the first five years of NHS England. London: The King's Fund; 2018.
9. Braithwaite J. Changing how we think about healthcare improvement. BMJ. 2018;361:k2014.
10. Greenhalgh T, Wherton J, Papoutsi C, et al. Beyond adoption: a new framework for theorizing and evaluating non-adoption, abandonment and challenges to the scale-up, spread and sustainability of health and care technologies. J Med Internet Res. 2017;19(11):e367.
11. Benson T, Grieve G. Principles of health interoperability: FHIR HL7 and SNOMED CT. 4th ed. London: Springer; 2021.
12. Rogers E. Diffusion of innovations. 5th ed. New York: Free Press; 2003.
13. Betton V. Towards a digital ecology: NHS digital adoption through the COVID-19 looking glass. CRC Press 2022.

Using the Results

6

Background

The value of all data, including PROMs and PREMs, depends on it being used to improve health and care. This needs good data. This book is about data, what PROMs and PREMs to collect and how best to do it. But we also need to understand the results, always remembering garbage in is garbage out (GIGO).

Analysis in the healthcare services is variable, and often poor. As with most problems in healthcare the problem is complex, with human, technical, cultural and regulatory barriers. An investigation into the state of data analysis in the NHS in England made 40 specific improvement suggestions [1].

An obvious issue is the workforce. In the English NHS about 1% of staff are data analysts with a wide variety of skills, backgrounds, and capabilities. Ignoring part-time analysts, at one end we have people who specialise in a narrow range of skills, such as coding diagnoses and procedures in order to maximise revenue under existing payment arrangements. These people are often poorly qualified and paid. Then, we have more senior people involved in quality improvement, operations research and similar disciplines. At the top end of the spectrum we find medical statisticians who design and analyse clinical trials, who often have a doctorate and links to a university.

Junior roles offer few opportunities for training, no professional development path, nor career trajectory. Analysis services require a new professional structure and substantial investment in training and education for both analysts and managers.

There is a further disconnect between analysts on one hand and managers and clinicians on the other. Some managers have little understanding of the limitations of the data available. As a result, they feel frustrated when the information they need is not available as required. Some also lack the data literacy and the statistical knowledge needed to conduct informed conversations about data.

© The Author(s), under exclusive license to Springer Nature Switzerland AG 2022
T. Benson, *Patient-Reported Outcomes and Experience*,
https://doi.org/10.1007/978-3-030-97071-0_6

Data analysts usually work within healthcare organizations without any external audit. The lack of professional structure, status and central support has led to a dearth of academic courses. For example, a search of the UCAS (Universities and Colleges Admissions Service for the UK) website found only 6 providers offer undergraduate courses starting in 2022 for *Health Informatics* (or similar terms). In comparison 81 providers offer courses for *Microbiology* and 240 for *Computer Games* [2]. The idea that this can be dealt with by post-graduate education does not wash. What is an appropriate first degree? The digital health field is far too broad for anyone to learn enough to be competent in just one year, let alone in a single module.

Most analysts use nothing more sophisticated than a spreadsheet. Spreadsheets are useful but notoriously error-prone. Anyone, who has tried to adapt a complex spreadsheet written by someone else, will know that they are a nightmare to change or adapt [3]. Medical statisticians use professional statistics tools, such as SPSS, SAS or R, but these tools expect users to understand exactly what they are doing. There are few good tools for less experienced staff.

In practice, most users of PROMs and PREMs do not see themselves as analysts but as managers or clinicians, although suppliers need to meet the needs of analysts and statisticians with strong analytical skills.

Analysis

Terms such as portal, analytics, business intelligence, performance dashboard and performance management have overlapping but distinct meanings. I use the word analysis as an umbrella term.

Roles

Different job roles use information in different ways.

Managers

Senior managers and leaders seek clear graphical trends for PROMs and PREMs to help them grasp what is happening and inform strategic decisions. Senior managers often have little time and want to see the conclusions as quickly as possible. They like charts, graphs and tables with colour codes (conditional formatting) to help them. At this level the focus is on monitoring and strategic decisions.

Junior managers like tables with supporting data, so that when they present summary results and recommendations to their superiors, they have more detailed data to back up their proposals. They are also likely to have operational responsibilities and want information that can help them in their daily work.

Analysts

Analysts need detailed information to help them understand what is happening at a group or cohort level. They are usually comfortable with summary tables, spreadsheets and statistics. They often need detailed data at the individual response level to back up their proposals. PROMs and PREMs data should be downloadable into comma separated variable (CSV) files for import into other packages.

Clinicians

Clinicians deal with individual patients and need detailed information to help them provide the best possible care at the individual level. They compare individual patients against their previous ratings and want to know if a change is clinically important or is noise or chance. Many clinicians also play other roles as well.

Most information users are casual users for whom understanding information is secondary to their primary job. They often have too much work to do already and some live in fear of being overwhelmed by too much data too often. But when a problem does arise, they want to see the full picture, so they can take appropriate action without delay.

People with limited ability to understand tables and charts may prefer a written interpretation, summarising the key points as narrative text.

Change

Working with PROMs and PREMs, the most common need is to measure improvement over time. The time interval varies with the type of intervention.

For surgical operations, such as total hip replacement, the key time interval may be several months (e.g., six months or a year) to allow the patient to recover. But even with surgery, it may be useful to measure more frequently to detect and treat post-operative infections and other complications. With non-invasive interventions, talking therapies or medication a shorter time frame (e.g., six weeks) is usually appropriate.

Another distinction is between time periods and individuals.

Time Period

If we want to look at all people seen during a particular period, we could compare all *before* measures done in the month with all *follow-up* measures done in the same month. However, this does not compare the same people and assumes that the two population groups have the same properties. This can be completely anonymous.

Period data solves the problem of how best to report one off visits, which do not lead to any treatment that needs to be followed up.

Individuals

If we look at the same people before and after, we can see their outcome on an individual basis. This is what most people imagine when they think about outcomes.

Taking the example of hip replacement, if the operation was done in May, with a follow up in November, the before and after comparison cannot be reported until 6 months after the operation. It needs a patient identifier to compare the same people. If a special-purpose identifier is used, or one provided by the patient and not shared with their clinicians, the patient can remain effectively anonymous.

Dashboard

A narrow definition of a dashboard is: *A visual display of the most important information needed to achieve one of more objectives; consolidated and arranged on a single screen so information can be monitored at a glanc* [4].

A broader definition is: *A layered information delivery system that parcels out information, insights and alerts to users on demand so that they can measure, monitor and manage business performance more effectively* [5].

The second definition omits the idea that everything must be on a single screen, and emphasises different layers of information for different user types. Both definitions focus on what people need to help them achieve specific objectives.

Dashboards can enable organisational change. Setting up a dashboard can help communicate strategy, show people how they will be judged and provide the opportunity to refine strategy in the light of what works best.

A dashboard can increase visibility into what is really happening. It is based on real-world data, aids communication between different departments, and helps ensure that is everyone is working to the same end. This increases motivation.

For this to work, the information needs to be relevant and easy to understand. In most cases this means being right up-to-date or at least cover the period up to the end of last month.

Dashboards for Managers

Managers use heuristics (quick rules of thumb) to monitor the performance over time. They assess the overall level and the direction of travel using a range of methods.

Scores

The first need for managers is a simple way to compare mean scores. It helps if all mean scores are displayed using the same scale and in the same direction. I like to use a scale from 0 to 100, where 0 represents the lowest possible mean score and 100 the highest possible.

If a measure comprises four items which are summed or averaged to produce a summary score, all mean scores can be transformed to a 0–100 scale, enabling simple comparison between item and summary scores.

It does not really matter what score you use, so long as all measures used are consistent. However, it is very confusing if a high score is good for one measure and bad for another measure. This should always be avoided.

Thresholds

Thresholds offer a simple type of comparison. The mean score is compared with predefined threshold values. A typical example of using thresholds is when the range of possible scores is divided into four classes, with thresholds defining the class boundaries.

Most of the measures described in this book are one-tailed measures, where a high sore is good, and indicates no problems. This data is naturally skewed (most people have few problems). For these I often use thresholds separating high (80–100), moderate (60–79), low (40–59) and very low (0–39) scores. Often, scores lying in these areas are colour-coded, such as green (80–100), yellow (60–79), orange (40–59) and red (0–39).

Another example comes from the Patient Activation Measure (PAM), where patients are allocated different levels (1–4) based on their answers.

Other measures, such as adult height, are normally distributed about a mean, with a two-tailed distribution; here standard deviations are often used as threshold at one standard deviation, two standard deviations and so on.

For example, the Physical Components Score (PCS) from SF-36 and SF-12 is based on a mean PCS = 50 and standard deviation of 10, based on a specific population sample. So, PCS = 40 is one standard deviation below the mean.

Periods

Time periods are frequently used as comparators. When monitoring performance, you may want to compare the mean scores for the most recent period of interest, which may be a month, quarter or year, with the long-term average or another period. This can be used to check on trends, rises or falls. This also gives the opportunity to check that the number of responses is in line with expectations.

Before and After

Other useful comparisons are between *before* and *after* scores, where change can also be seen. Change can also have its own thresholds, based on either statistical tests (such as 95% confidence limits) or predefined values (such as 10 points), which may be related to confidence limits.

Demographics

Demographic data provides additional contextual information. For many purposes a simple frequency count, combined with period analysis, is enough to show whether the survey population is changing. Filters may also be used.

Downloads

For more complex and ad hoc analysis it is usually cost-effective to download data as a CSV file for subsequent processing in a spreadsheet or statistics package. You can do a lot using a spreadsheet, such as Excel, but spreadsheets make it very hard for others to understand exactly what you have done.

Case Study

An example of a dashboard table from a social prescribing provider is shown as Table 6.1. The data shown is for 'linked' data, where we compare before and after results for the same patients. *Before* data refers to measures at first meeting after referral; *After* is six weeks later after weekly contacts.

This shows the results for four measures: Health status, Health confidence, Personal wellbeing and Patient experience. The first column shows each measure and its component items. These measures and items are described in more detail in Chaps. 10–13.

The next columns are shown in two groups of three. The first group shows the mean scores for the whole period July 2020 to December 2021, the second for the quarter, October 2021 to December 2021. In each group, the mean Before and After scores are shown on a scale from 0 to 100, plus the difference between them.

Table 6.1 Example of social prescribing dashboard table (© R-Outcomes Ltd. 2022).

Social Prescribing	Jul 20 - Dec 21			Oct 21 - Dec 21		
Measure	Before	After	Diff	Before	After	Diff
Health Status	54	71	+17*	52	73	+21**
	(n353)	(n358)		(n75)	(n75)	
Pain or discomfort	69	77	+8	68	76	+8
Feeling low or worried	40	69	+29**	44	71	+27**
Limited in what you can do	50	68	+18*	46	73	+27**
Require help from others	56	70	+14*	52	74	+22**
Health Confidence	61	80	+19*	58	81	+23**
	(n354)	(n353)		(n74)	(n74)	
I know enough about my health	59	76	+17*	57	76	+19*
I can look after my health	56	74	+18*	54	76	+22**
I can get the right help if I need it	57	81	+24**	55	82	+27**
I am involved in decisions about me	73	90	+17*	67	90	+23**
Personal Wellbeing	40	63	+23**	42	63	+21**
	(n355)	(n354)		(n75)	(n74)	
I am satisfied with my life	42	65	+23**	46	65	+19*
What I do in my life is worthwhile	46	67	+21**	47	68	+21**
I was happy yesterday	39	63	+24**	40	60	+20**
I was NOT anxious yesterday	32	58	+26**	36	59	+23**
Patient Experience	68	74	+6	67	78	+11*
	(n281)	(n346)		(n49)	(n75)	
Treat me kindly	69	74	+5	69	79	+10*
Listen and explain	68	74	+6	67	78	+11*
See me promptly	68	73	+5	65	77	+12*
Well organised	68	74	+6	67	78	+11*

n refers to the number of responses.
* indicates a change of 10 to 20;
** indicates a change of over 20.

Improvements of more than 10 points are indicated with one star, over 20 points with two stars.

Conditional formatting is used to highlight scores in bands: red 0–39, orange 40–59, yellow 60–79, green over 80.

Readers should note the values of each item as well as the amount of improvement (difference). It is easier to improve an item that starts at a low value, than one that starts at a high value. For example, personal wellbeing before scores are much lower scores than patient experience before scores. Personal wellbeing improves much more, but the after scores are still lower than the patient experience after scores, which have shown less improvement. For these scores any improvement of more than 5 points is likely to be important.

The number of responses for each measure is also shown such as (n353). If the number of responses is very low (less than 5), comparisons are not reliable.

Statistical Packages

Many statistics packages are available. The leading tools have been under continuous development for over 50 years. They fall into two main groups: proprietary and free open-source.

The leading proprietary products are SAS, Stata and SPSS. These are comprehensive, complex, and expensive. They expect users to know exactly what they are doing.

The leading free open-source package is R. This is also comprehensive and complex.

R has several graphical front ends, which are relatively straightforward to use. I use JASP, which is developed at the University of Amsterdam and has an intuitive user interface [6]. JASP has been used for all the statistical calculations in this book.

Once you have found a package that you like and know how to use effectively, there is no incentive to move to different one, unless that is what your employer requires you to do.

Advanced statistical analysis is beyond the scope of this book. A good starting point is Streiner, Norman and Cairney [7].

Validity

Any test or measure may be valid for one purpose but not for another. The process of validation involves assembling evidence and arguments that support validity for a specific purpose. All too often PROMs and PREMs are re-used for purposes other than the purpose for which they were originally designed and validated.

The authoritative *Standards for Educational and Psychological Testing* defines validity as follows [8]:

Validity refers to the degree to which evidence and theory support the interpretation of test scores for the proposed uses of tests. Validity is therefore the most fundamental consideration in developing tests and evaluation tests. The process of evaluation involves accumulating relevant evidence to provide a sound scientific basis for the proposed score interpretations. It is the interpretations of test scores for proposed uses that are evaluated, not the test itself. ... It is incorrect to use the unqualified phrase "the validity of the test."

Construct Validation

Construct validity is the degree to which a test measures what it claims or purports to be measuring. This is the overarching concern in validity and subsumes all other types of validity evidence. Key to construct validity are the theoretical ideas behind what is being considered. Often constructs, such as experience or well-being, cannot be measured directly and unambiguously, but have multiple aspects, which can be measured separately.

Several types of evidence are used in construct validation, such as:

1. Content—does the wording, format and scoring appear to be measuring the construct of interest?
2. Response process—do respondents interpret the items in the way that the designer intended, as measured against the intended construct?
3. Internal structure—do item interrelationships conform with the intended construct?
4. Relations with other variables—are patterns of relationships between test scores and other variables as predicted by the intended construct?
5. Consequences—can intended and unintended results can be traced back to the measure?

Other Types of Validity

Other types of validity include criterion validity and content validity.

Criterion validity looks at correlations between the results and other variables that measure the same thing. It depends on there being a suitable criterion.

Content validity is an informal assessment of whether the measure covers the main constructs described in the literature. It is related to face validity, although face validity is even less rigorous and may be based on amateur opinion.

Example

An easy way to explore the requirements is through an example.

Mary manages a small team which provides a physiotherapy with weekly appointments for patients who are referred to it. For two years the team has collected health status data on each patient on referral and at the end of the intervention six weeks later.

Each month Mary gets a report where she checks the following things:

- How many patients have been referred to us in the last month? Is this higher or lower than expected?
- Are patients referred last month any different in terms of health status from those usually seen over the past two years? If so, are they better or worse?
- Have patients got better, and by how much? Is this more or less than usual?
- Are the results for any items (questions) in different from the others? If so, why?
- Does the summary score accurately represent what is going on? Does it agree with what staff tell me?

This leads to the following requirements:

- Show before, after and difference numbers and scores.
- Show last month and all-time numbers and scores.
- Indicate whether scores and changes are above or below various thresholds.

Mary also uses this data to support a bid for more staff, by showing that her workload has increased, the average severity of patients being referred has become worse, and her outcomes have begun to suffer.

Publication Check-List

The ISPOR Consolidated Health Economic Evaluation Reporting Standards (CHEERS) task force has developed a 28-point check-list for how heath economic studies should be reported in the academic literature. Only a few items (identified) are applicable only to economics studies (see Table 6.2) [9].

Table 6.2 CHEERS checklist for health economic evaluations [9]

No	Section/topic	Guidance for reporting
1	Title	Identify the study as an (economic) evaluation and specify the interventions being compared
2	Abstract	Provide a structured summary that highlights context, key methods, results, and alternative analyses
3	Background and objectives	Give the context for the study, the study question, and its practical relevance for decision making in policy or practice
Methods		
4	Health economic analysis plan	Indicate whether a (health economic) analysis plan was developed and where available
5	Study population	Describe characteristics of the study population (such as age range, demographics, socioeconomic, or clinical characteristics)

(continued)

Table 6.2 (continued)

No	Section/topic	Guidance for reporting
6	Setting and location	Provide relevant contextual information that may influence findings
7	Comparators	Describe the interventions or strategies being compared and why chosen
8	Perspective	State the perspective(s) adopted by the study and why chosen
9	Time horizon	State the time horizon for the study and why appropriate
10	Discount rate	Report the discount rate(s) and reason chosen (for economics studies)
11	Selection of outcomes	Describe what outcomes were used as the measure(s) of benefit(s) and harm(s)
12	Measurement of outcomes	Describe how outcomes used to capture benefit(s) and harm(s) were measured
13	Valuation of outcomes	Describe the population and methods used to measure and value outcomes
14	Measurement and valuation of resources and costs	Describe how costs were valued (for economics studies)
15	Currency, price date, and conversion	Report the dates of the estimated resource quantities and unit costs, plus the currency and year of conversion (for economics studies)
16	Rationale and description of model	If modeling is used, describe in detail and why used. Report if the model is publicly available and where it can be accessed
17	Analytics and assumptions	Describe any methods for analysing or statistically transforming data, any extrapolation methods, and approaches for validating any model used
18	Characterizing heterogeneity	Describe any methods used for estimating how the results of the study vary for subgroups
19	Characterizing distributional effects	Describe how impacts are distributed across different individuals or adjustments made to reflect priority populations
20	Characterizing uncertainty	Describe methods to characterize any sources of uncertainty in the analysis
21	Approach to engagement with patients and others affected by the study	Describe any approaches to engage patients or service recipients, the general public, communities, or stakeholders (such as clinicians or payers) in the design of the study
Results		
22	Study parameters	Report all analytic inputs (such as values, ranges, references) including uncertainty or distributional assumptions
23	Summary of main results	Report the mean values for the main categories of costs and outcomes of interest and summarize them in the most appropriate overall measure

(continued)

Table 6.2 (continued)

No	Section/topic	Guidance for reporting
24	Effect of uncertainty	Describe how uncertainty about analytic judgments, inputs, or projections affect findings. Report the effect of choice of discount rate and time horizon, if applicable
25	Effect of engagement with patients and others affected by the study	Report on any difference patient/service recipient, general public, community, or stakeholder involvement made to the approach or findings of the study
Discussion		
26	Study findings, limitations, generalizability, and current knowledge	Report key findings, limitations, ethical or equity considerations not captured, and how these could affect patients, policy, or practice
Other		
27	Source of funding	Describe how the study was funded and any role of the funder in the identification, design, conduct, and reporting of the analysis
28	Conflicts of interest	Report authors' conflicts of interest according to journal or International Committee of Medical Journal Editors requirements

Conclusions

Analysis and the presentation of results is a key requirement for PROMs and PREMs.

Much needs to be done to improve the status of analysts within the healthcare services. Spreadsheets are capable but hard to support and maintain.

Different user roles need to know different things. Dashboards provide a useful way to show information that can be readily understood.

Statistics packages are needed for more advanced uses such as validation studies.

References

1. Goldacre B, Bardsley M, Benson T, et al. Bringing NHS data analysis into the 21st century. J R Soc Med. 2020;113(10):383–8.
2. UCAS (Universities and Colleges Admissions Service). https://www.ucas.com. Accessed 30 October 2021.
3. Caulkins J, Morrison E, Weidemann T. Spreadsheet errors and decision making: evidence from field interviews. J Organ End User Comput (JOEUC). 2007;19(3):1–23.
4. Few S. Information dashboard design: the effective visual communication of data. North Sebastopol CA: O'Reilly; 2006.
5. Eckerson W. Performance dashboards: measuring, monitoring and managing your business. 2nd ed. Hoboken NJ: Wiley; 2011.
6. JASP Team. JASP Version 0.16. 2021 [Computer software].

7. Streiner DL, Norman GR, Cairney J. Health measurement scales: a practical guide to their development and use. 5th ed. Oxford University Press; 2015.
8. American Educational Research Association, American Psychological Association, National Council on Measurement in Education (eds). Standards for educational and psychological testing. Lanham MD: American Educational Research Association; 2014.
9. Husereau D, Drummond M, Augustovski F, et al. Consolidated health economic evaluation reporting standards (CHEERS) 2022 explanation and elaboration: a report of the ISPOR CHEERS II good practices task force. Value Health. 2022;25(1):10–31.

Sharing Data 7

What Is Interoperability

Interoperability enables information to be shared with and re-used by others, reducing the need for duplicated effort. It is one of the keys to making healthcare more cost-effective.

A full chapter about interoperability is unusual in a book about PROMs and PREMs, but it is one of the key missing pieces of the jigsaw. This chapter only provides a simple introduction to healthcare interoperability, which is quite complex. To learn more, see *Principles of Health Interoperability FHIR HL7 and SNOMED CT* [1].

One definition of interoperability is *the ability of two or more systems or components to exchange information and to use the information that has been exchanged* [2].

There are for main types of interoperability: technical, semantic, process and clinical.

Technical Interoperability

Technical interoperability is the ability to move data from A to B without error. This is domain-independent and is based on information theory, which was originally developed during the second World War [3]. This is now a standard commodity. For example, the Internet depends on technical interoperability.

Semantic Interoperability

Semantic interoperability is the exchange of meaning between two systems. This depends on system A and system B understanding data in the same way. It is domain-specific. Systems used in banking do not semantically interoperate with those used in healthcare. Healthcare interoperability standards focus on semantic interoperability. It needs agreed codes and identifiers.

Process Interoperability

Process interoperability is when operational systems at A and B work together. It is process- and context-specific. Process interoperability can enable great savings in efficiency but requires substantial investment in business process re-engineering and staff training.

Clinical Interoperability

Clinical interoperability is when two or more clinicians in different care teams can transfer patients between them and provide seamless care to patients. This is what we all need. Unfortunately, it seldom happens because it depends on technical, semantic and process interoperability all working perfectly.

Layers of Interoperability

Another way to think of interoperability is in layers: technology, data, human and institution.

Technology Layer

The technology layer is the technical nuts and bolts of how information is exchanged in a way that is safe and reliable. This is where HL7 FHIR standards and application program interfaces (APIs) belong.

Data Layer

The data layer deals with the exchange of meaning and needs standardized identifiers and codes such as SNOMED CT and LOINC.

Human Layer

The human layer is where people get involved. This covers re-engineered clinical and administrative processes, training and support.

Institutional Layer

The institutional layer is about incentives and penalties. Standards, information governance, culture and regulation play important key roles in creating or removing barriers to interoperability.

Some of the human and institutional issues have been discussed in Chaps. 4 and 5.

Interoperability Standards

A standard is defined as:

> A document, established by consensus and approved by a recognized body (such as an accredited standards development organization), that provides, for common and repeated

use, rules, guidelines, or characteristics for activities or their results, aimed at the optimum degree of order in a given context.

Consensus is general agreement, characterized by the absence of sustained opposition to substantial issues by any important part of the concerned interests and by a process that involves seeking to take into account the views of all parties concerned and to reconcile any conflicting arguments. Consensus need not imply unanimity [4].

Healthcare interoperability standards aim to enable safe, efficient, and effective care by helping to deliver the right information at the right place at the right time for the right people.

Why Interoperability Is Hard

Healthcare is complex and the number of people who need to be kept up to date can be surprisingly large, especially if patients have multiple conditions. The number of links needed to keep N people up to date increases with as N squared. The actual formula is $(N^2 - N)/2$.

The cost of developing a single bespoke interface is less than that of developing a standards-based interface, but each new interface costs roughly the same. Standards-based interfaces have a higher initial cost, but each subsequent one is much cheaper. The basic economics are illustrated in Fig. 7.1.

Standards simplify communications between multiple parties as shown in Fig. 7.2. Other benefits of using interoperability standards include the multiplier effect, where the more they are used the more benefits you get, and avoidance of supplier lock-in giving customers more choice, competition and flexibility. Some suppliers consider this is a threat.

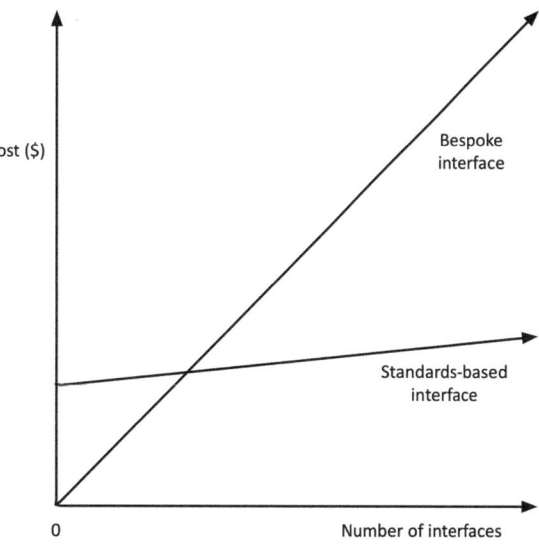

Fig. 7.1 Interoperability economics

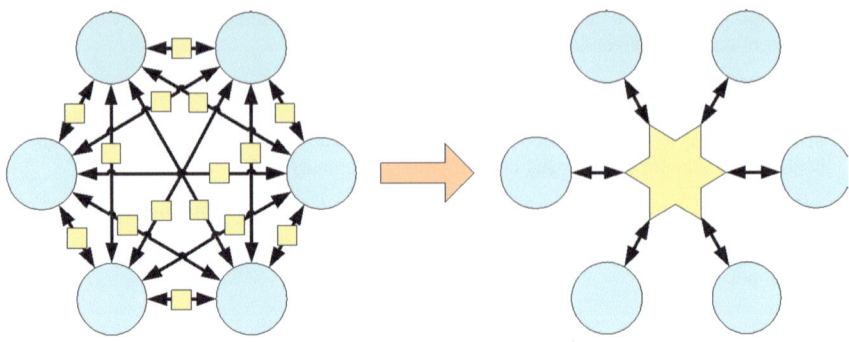

Fig. 7.2 The way that a standard can simplify communication

Computers hate ambiguity, but natural language is often ambiguous and context-specific. To exchange information between two or more computers needs a specialised unambiguous language, which is understood by both sender and receiver systems.

All languages have syntax, protocols, terms and identifiers. Syntax is the formal rules of a language, the grammar. Today, the best language to use is HL7 FHIR R4 (see below), but there are other options. Protocols or interactions specify what can be done, how, and in what order. Terms are words or phrases used to describe a thing or concept in a particular context. Identifiers are labels or names of things or concepts. In computer interoperability identifiers must be unique.

Interoperability is notoriously hard. This is because software developers for every application use their own computer specific dialect within their systems. The sender needs to translate this dialect for their own users, who usually speak their own specialty-specific medical dialect and also into the language used in interoperability, such as HL7 FHIR. The developers at the receiving system have to do the reverse and translate HL7 FHIR into their own native dialect and for their own users, who usually speak a slightly different medical dialect. Each of these translations needs to be perfect because computers are digital and do not tolerate errors.

HL7 FHIR

HL7 FHIR (Fast Health Interoperability Resources, pronounced "fire") has become the internationally accepted way to exchange information between computer applications in healthcare [5].

FHIR is Release 4 (R4), was issued in 2020 and has been endorsed at government level in many countries, including USA and UK. Future releases are expected to be backward compatible with FHIR R4. It is widely expected that FHIR will drive the costs of interoperability down, while increasing expectations and the overall spend on integration.

FHIR is still young. The core ideas were first proposed by Grahame Grieve in 2011, based on ideas that were already proving successful in web-based applications such as social media. The key ideas are outlined in the FHIR manifesto:

- Focus on implementers; all specifications come with examples and reference implementations.
- Target support for common scenarios that are widely needed and used.
- Leverage standard cross-industry web technologies such as REST, JSON, HTTPS and OAuth.
- Require human readability along with codes as a base level of interoperability.
- Make content freely available; all FHIR materials are free of charge.
- Support multiple paradigms and architectures including APIs, messaging and document exchange.
- Demonstrate best practice governance.

RESTful APIs

FHIR is based on the ideas of REST (Representational state transfer) originally developed by Roy Fielding [6]. The term RESTful means that the interface is based on REST but may not be 100% compliant with other RESTful specifications. RESTful interfaces, such as FHIR, conform to five principles:

- Resources are identified using URLs (uniform interface).
- Client and server are separate (client/server).
- No client context is stored on the server between requests (stateless interactions).
- Responses can be cached.
- The client does not know whether it is talking to the server or an intermediary (layered).

Most FHIR implementations are APIs (application program interfaces) or webhooks (called Resource Subscriptions in FHIR), but FHIR can be used for messaging and document exchange applications too.

APIs enable two-way communications between software applications based on requests for information and responses. Webhooks are light-weight APIs that enable one-way sending of information when an event takes place. This is an active development area in FHIR.

The core FHIR standard is too general to be used as is. All implementations use FHIR Profiles, which specify exactly what is needed to do specific tasks in specified places. FHIR Profiles also specify the terminology bindings, which say what terms shall be used in each situation. Usually terminology bindings select codes from comprehensive terminology systems such as SNOMED CT and LOINC (see below).

There are many other security and safety issues.

Structured Data

Structured data is ubiquitous in health care, with many applications for patients, clinicians and administrative staff.

Patients complete questionnaires with their medical, family and social history and eligibility criteria, as well as for quality improvement, evaluation and monitoring of outcomes and experience of care (PROMs and PREMs) [7].

Clinicians use assessments and questionnaires to ensure that they conform to best practice, for audit, computer-based decision support and to automatically encode data as they work. It is quicker and easier to click a box than to look up codes as you work.

Administrative work involves completing and using questionnaires and forms. Researchers, public health and payers also need standardised data.

Some questionnaires and forms, such as referrals templates, test requests and admission forms are already standardized in most institutions. In other scenarios data is collected using user-defined screens and forms.

Before describing specific FHIR resources, we outline a couple of use cases involving PROMs and PREMs where interoperability is useful.

Use Cases

A use case is a list of actions or event steps typically defining the interactions between a role and a system to achieve some goal. The role can be played by a human or a computer.

Notifications

Notifications are commonly used throughout the health and care system to tell others that something has happened. For example, when someone is discharged from hospital, this may be the trigger to send them a PROMs/PREMs survey. However, if they died, no survey should be sent now or in future.

Often notification is much more efficiently done computer-to-computer than using human intermediaries. If humans are involved, the sender must be notified and prepare and send the notification; this is then sent to the receiver who opens and processes it. Errors can occur at every stage. Using computer interoperability, these systems can be streamlined, eliminating errors and tasks for people at both sender and receiver ends.

The amount of information contained in a notification is often small, typically no more than who, what, when and where. It needs to happen immediately a trigger event takes place. This is the sort of thing that Webhooks are designed for.

Data update

Data update, such as importing PROMs/PREMs results may be done at regular intervals or on demand. For example, a patient portal may be updated with each day's results every night, or a clinician may want to see the latest results for a patient. This uses a request-response mechanism. The requester (client) sends out a request for particular information and the server responds accordingly.

Data update is more complicated than simple notification, because the sequence of messages is more complicated and there is a lot more data involved. This is what conventional APIs do.

FHIR Resources

FHIR Resources are the basic building blocks of FHIR. To date about 150 resources have been defined, organised into five main groups: Foundation, Base, Clinical, Financial and Specialized. Each group has a further 4 or 5 categories, to assist finding the one you need.

All FHIR resources have a narrative part, defined structured data and optional extensions to meet local needs. Message profiles usually include multiple resources. For example, a laboratory report includes results data and also information about the patient, laboratory and requester.

FHIR provides two resources to support PROMs and PREMs, focused on the question and answer paradigm:

- Questionnaire: the design of the form, with the questions to answer (empty). This is a specialised definitional artifact resource. This is not used as much as the QestionnaireResponse resource.
- QuestionnaireResponse: a set of answers to the questions from a person (completed). This is a clinical diagnostics resource.

Questionnaire and QuestionnaireResponse resources provide the basic structures used by all applications where forms are used.

The FHIR community has collaborated on an implementation guide called *Structured Data Capture* (SDC) which builds on the base questionnaire resource by specifying extensions, profiles, operations, and services to support:

- Pre-populating questionnaires with answers already known to the system
- Full control over how the questionnaires are presented
- Support for answers with calculated scores and conditional questions
- Fully adaptive forms which start empty and are driven by AI backend systems.

The SDC guide aims to: save time by preventing clinicians from feeling like expensive clerical workers; to improve data quality, by enabling checks and validating responses; and use data for comparisons over time and between groups [8].

Questionnaire

A Questionnaire (sometimes abbreviated to Q) is an organized collection of questions intended to solicit information from patients, providers or other individuals involved in the healthcare domain. Questionnaires may be simple flat lists of questions or hierarchically organized in groups and sub-groups, each containing questions. Questionnaire defines the questions to be asked, how they are ordered and grouped, any intervening instructional text and constraints on the allowed answers. The result of filling out a Questionnaire with a set of answers is communicated using the *QuestionnaireResponse* resource (see below).

Questionnaires define the specifics about data capture—exactly what questions are asked, in what order, what choices for answers are, etc. Questionnaire is a separately identifiable resource, but individual questions are not.

Questionnaire is focused on user-facing data collection. For each question it includes information such as what number or label should be displayed beside each question, conditions in which questions should be displayed (or not), what instructions should be provided to the user and so on.

Questionnaire Content

The Questionnaire resource contains information (metadata) about the questionnaire itself, and a series of nested *items* which may be labels, questions, or groups of other questions. Each Questionnaire contains at least one Item (question). Items can repeat and/or nest using sub-items.

Answers may be linked to terminologies. Items may have any number of specified AnswerOptions, which are the possible answers. Each item within a Questionnaire has a *linkId* uniquely identifying it. This is used to link the question to the response in the QuestionnaireResponse. Other elements within each item may provide detailed formatting instructions and user hints.

The questionnaire item types supported are shown in Table 7.1

Other classes cover Initial or default values and EnableWhen instructions, such as branching based on previous answers (Fig. 7.3).

QuestionnaireResponse

A QuestionnaireResponse (sometimes abbreviated to QR) contains a set of answers submitted to the questions in questionnaire. The answers are ordered and grouped into coherent subsets, corresponding to the structure of the questions in the Questionnaire being responded to.

In addition, the QuestionnaireResponse contains minimal information about the questions—the *linkId* that refers back to the question in the matching Questionnaire, and text of the question so that the answers can be displayed without having to retrieve the source questionnaire.

Table 7.1 Questionnaire item type value set[1]

Item type	Definition
group	An item with children, may be repeating. Could be a section, table or other layout
display	Just a label to be displayed (no answer to be collected)
boolean	Yes/no answer (checkbox, radio group or similar)
decimal	Real number answer
integer	Integer answer
date	Date answer
dateTime	Date and time answer
time	Time only answer (hour: minute: second) answer independent of date
string	Short free-text answer
text	Longer free-text answer, potentially multi-paragraph (multi-line textbox)
url	URL (website, FTP site, etc.) answer (restricted textbox)
Coding	Coding—generally drawn from a list of possible answers (valueCoding) as an answer
attachment	Binary content such as a image, PDF, etc. as an answer
reference	A reference to another resource, e.g. practitioner, organization, etc
quantity	Question with a combination of a numeric value and unit

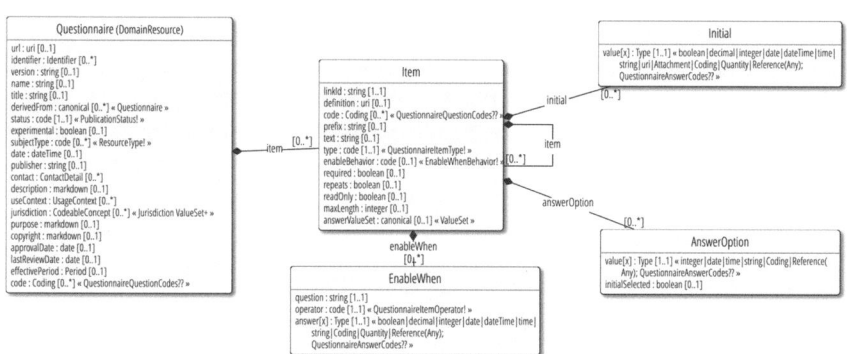

Fig. 7.3 FHIR Questionnaire resource UML diagram

Each time a questionnaire is completed for a different subject or at a different time, a separate QuestionnaireResponse is generated, although it is also possible for a previously entered set of answers to be edited or updated.

---

[1] see http://hl7.org/fhir/valueset-item-type.html.

QuestionnaireResponse covers the need to communicate data originating from forms used in medical history examinations, research questionnaires and even full clinical specialty records. In many systems this data is collected using user-defined screens and forms.

QuestionnaireResponse records specifics about data capture—what questions were asked, in what order, what answers were given, etc. QuestionnaireResponse is a separately identifiable resource, whereas the individual answers are not.

QuestionnaireResponse may not refer to a Questionnaire on which it is based. If it does, it can be validated to verify that required groups and questions are answered and that answers fit constraints in terms of cardinality, data type, etc. In particular, the Item *linkId*s must match, as must the order and any nesting.

The order of questions is relevant within groups, groups within groups and groups within questions and must be retained for display and capture. The hierarchy items within the QuestionnaireResponse must mirror the hierarchy of the corresponding Questionnaire (if any).

QuestionnaireResponse Content

The QuestionnaireResponse has a similar shape to the Questionnaire resource. The main QuestionnaireResponse class may have any number of child Item classes, which in turn may have any number of Answer classes. Items and Answers can be nested or repeated, if required (Fig. 7.4).

Questionnaire responses can be authored by clinicians, patients, or patients' relatives (or even owners in the case of animals). Clinicians may author questionnaire responses as a proxy, where the answers are provided by others on behalf of the patient. Additionally, information gathered on behalf of a patient may be about the patient's relatives (e.g. family history). Therefore, QuestionnaireResponse makes a distinction between the *author*, *source of information* and *subject*. Any of these can be a person (Practitioner, Patient or RelatedPerson). In addition, *author*

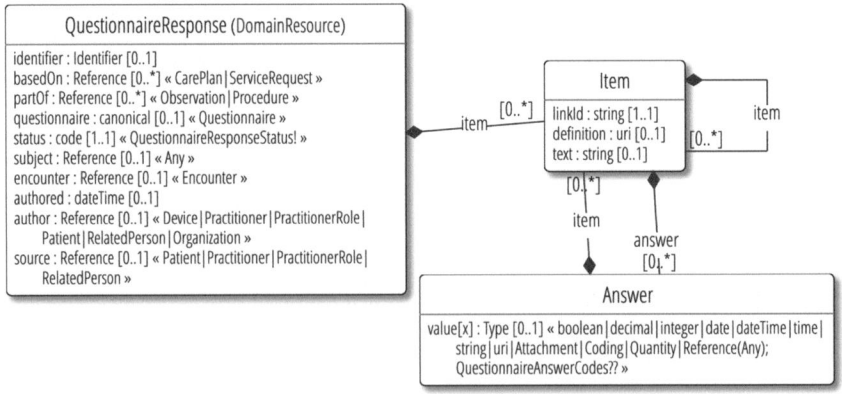

Fig. 7.4 FHIR QuestionnaireResponse resource UML diagram

could be a Device or Organization and the *subject* could be person, organization, animal, thing or even a place.

QuestionnaireResponse can be used to capture any type of data, including data that would typically map to other FHIR resources. Data types can be a primitive data type such as boolean (Yes/No), decimal, integer, date, dateTime, time, string, uri, or a complex data type such as attachment, coding, quantity or reference.

The focus of QuestionnaireResponse includes the specific phrasing and organization of the questions. All data are captured as question and answer.

The QuestionnaireResponse *encounter* element can be used to link to the encounter when the questionnaire response was authored. This may be relevant since the encounter gives context to the answers and can be used to relate information in the QuestionnaireResponse to orders and observations done during the same encounter.

Relationships with Other Resources

Questionnaire and QuestionnaireResponse can include data that could be represented using other resources. In fact, it usually does. Most of the information that is in a Questionnaire could be represented using the Observation resource.

The general pattern is that data is collected/captured using a Questionnaire, and the responses are stored as a QuestionnaireResponse but useful data from the answers may also be published using generated resources, especially observations.

Not all answers in a questionnaire are useful beyond the questionnaire itself. For example, "Do you have any symptoms of COVID-19?" is important as an observation, but "Have any other symptoms increased recently?" is probably not meaningful outside the questionnaire itself.

To help with managing this relationship, an item in a Questionnaire can have a series of codes associated with it. When codes are present, the questionnaire item can automatically be turned into an observation using that code. The answer can also be prepopulated if an observation already exists in the patient record with the right code. The SDC guide defines an extension that indicates how long an existing observation is valid (e.g. some vital signs are generally only valid for minutes, while others may be valid for months or years).

QuestionnaireResponse resources may also include data found in other resources. In these cases, the relationship between the question/answer and the underlying resources is more complex; the SDC specification defines a framework for locating pre-existing data and extracting the data from a set of questions into other resources.

Workflow

The SDC workflow has identified the following distinct computer system roles (Table 7.2):

Table 7.2 System roles with questionnaire

System role	Description
Form Designer	System responsible for creating and editing form designs
Form Filler	System responsible for capturing user form input to produce partially or fully completed forms
Form Manager	Repository for form definitions. May also perform pre-population
Form Response Manager	Searchable repository for storage and retrieval of completed and partially completed forms
Form Receiver	Write-only destination to which forms are sent for processing
Form Archiver	Write-only system responsible for archiving completed forms as well as works in progress

In this context a form is a questionnaire. In some cases one system may carry out several of these roles and not all of the roles are always needed. For example, the respondent will usually only see the Form Filler.

In form curation, the Form Designer interacts with both the Form Manager and a Data Element Registry to create, edit and update forms, including identifying and defining associated terminologies and data elements. This is an iterative process where an initial version is created and then subsequently updated and maintained, eventually changing status to active and later retired.

The more significant (and complex) workflow in SDC is to complete (and potentially submit) a completed questionnaire response.

The driver of this workflow is the Form Filler system. It retrieves a form (Questionnaire) from the Form Manager. It may also request that the Form Manager generate an initial QuestionnaireResponse, potentially partially populated with information known by the Form Manager, supplied by the Form Filler or queried from an underlying EHR. The Form Filler could generate the QuestionnaireResponse itself without the assistance of the Form Manager and in either case could partially fill in the response based on information known by the Form Filler.

When as much of the questionnaire response as possible has been filled in by automated means, the form is displayed to an end-user who reviews and edits the automatically populated content and completes those portions of the form that were not populated automatically. In the case of surveys this will be most of the form. In some cases, the form may be stored locally or using a Form Response Manager to allow a user to stop and resume editing at a later point.

The Form Filler (possibly with help from the Form Manager) is responsible for verifying that a completed form is complete and valid against the corresponding Questionnaire. Once valid, the Form Filler submits the form to one or more target repositories (Form Receiver allows the completed form to be subsequently retrieved, but Form Archiver does not) and/or stores the completed form itself. (Note—Form Receivers may perform validation on forms prior to consumption, Form Archivers typically will not.) The receiver of the completed form might then extract the data into relevant FHIR resources.

Most day-to-day questionnaires have a simpler workflow than that described above, but this illustrates the capability of the system. In theory, it should be possible to automate the entire user interface for data collection in an EHR using SDC driven data forms, but no one has tried this yet, so the FHIR Community doesn't know whether that's possible, or even whether that should be an explicit goal.

Static Forms

The most common implementation uses a static form or survey (the preliminary stage of authoring and distributing the Questionnaire is excluded).

This has the following lifecycle, focusing on what the systems do:

1. Select or trigger an existing questionnaire to use. This may be done automatically in response to a trigger event or be instigated by a clinician.
2. Load/render questionnaire (including referenced content such as code sets).
3. Optionally, pre-populate questionnaire with other data (such as patient demographics, past findings etc.) before displaying it to the end user. This saves users time by completing all information items that the system already knows.
4. User enters data.
5. Save QuestionnaireResponse, validate (with possible errors/warnings/issues reported back to the user), calculate any summary scores, etc.
6. Extract data into other FHIR resources for further use and analysis.
7. Later on, locate and fetch QuestionnaireResponse for review, data aggregation, analysis etc.

Not all of these steps will be needed for many implementations. This list excludes what is done with the results, because this differs depending on the use case.

From the user's point of view, they simply fill in the form and expect it to be checked and saved.

FHIR Search functions return complete QuestionnaireResponse resources. Individual answers to Questionnaire Items are not directly searchable using the FHIR API, because they are often context specific. To search individual responses, they must be converted to a more searchable form such as an EPR or FHIR Observations.

Computerized Adaptive Testing

Adaptive questionnaires are dynamic forms that adjust what questions are asked based on previous answers. This is also known as Computerized Adaptive Testing (CAT). The logic to determine the questions is defined external to the Questionnaire resource.

CATs are a type of measure in which the questions a person answers are based on their previous responses. Most CATs begin from an item bank, which is a collection of items (questions) all measuring the same thing (e.g. physical function). Items are ordered by level of difficulty/severity from low (e.g. I have difficulty getting in and out of bed) to high (I am able to run 5 miles) using Item Response Theory.

The first item administered in a CAT is usually one in the middle of the range of function or symptom severity. After a person provides a response, an estimated score is calculated. The CAT algorithm then selects the best item in the item bank for refining the estimated score. After a person provides a response, the estimated score is recalculated. The CAT continues to administer items until a limit is reached, which may be a specified level of measurement precision or simply a number of items asked.

In FHIR, the CAT is treated as a black box. The main difference between CAT and static forms is that the workflow is more complex—after answering each question, the form filler sends the current questionnaire response containing all the patient's responses to this point to the CAT service to find out what the next question should be using the $next-question operation.

Coding Schemes

Coded terms are essential in health interoperability to minimise ambiguity.

LOINC and SNOMED CT are two terminology systems have been developed to help semantic interoperability [9]. Examples of LOINC and SNOMED CT codes for some of the measures described in Part II of this book are shown in Appendix 1.

LOINC

LOINC (Logical Observation Identifiers Names and Codes) was designed specifically to support interoperability. LOINC was set up in 1994 and is free of charge [10].

The overall scope of LOINC is anything you can test, measure, or observe about a patient. LOINC codes represent the names of observations as opposed to the content of specific patient records. Think of an observation as the question, and the observation result as the answer. For example, LOINC might have a code of *eye colour*. An findings for a specific patient (e.g. *brown eyes*) may be coded using SNOMED CT.

LOINC distinguishes observations, such as tests ordered, survey questions or clinical documents, using six dimensions. The example is the LOINC representation of the howRu health status measure score described in Chap. 11.

1. Component—what is being measured or observed (e.g., howRu score).
2. Property—the characteristic or attribute of the component (e.g., Score).
3. Time—the time interval over which an observation is made (e.g., Pt). Pt means point in time.
4. System—what the observation is about (e.g., ^Patient).

Coding Schemes

5. Scale—whether the observation is nominal, ordinal, or quantitative (e.g., Qn). Qn means quantitative.
6. Method—this is optional to classify how the observation was made (e.g., howRu).

LOINC specifies a code and three names for every observation:

1. Code (55749–6). This is meaningless and includes a check digit after the hyphen.
2. Detailed fully specified name (FSN) based on the six dimensions above (e.g., howRu score:Score:Pt:^Patient:Qn:howRu)
3. User friendly long common name (LCN) (e.g., howRu score)
4. Short name, used on column headings (e.g., howRu score).

Survey items also have answer lists, which specify all possible options. These have special LOINC codes and attributes for what is shown to the responder and for scoring. These answer lists can be reused across multiple surveys. Examples of an answer list might be: *blue eyes*, *brown eyes*, *green eyes* etc. Note that the answer list is a property of the survey, not of the respondent.

At first sight LOINC looks complicated, partly because it has many codes which only differ in one small way from each other. This is needed to ensure that meaning is unambiguous. However, LOINC does what it says it does, and it is relatively quick and easy to add new codes.

SNOMED CT

SNOMED CT was released initially in 2002 and is regularly updated. It is large and relatively complex. It is intended to provide an extendible foundation for expressing clinical data about patients in electronic patient records, for interoperability and to support analysis and clinical decision support applications. It has three main component types: *concepts*, *descriptions,* and *relationships* [11].

All components have a SNOMED CT identifier (*sctId*), which is unique, numeric and machine readable, with no human-interpretable meaning. This is between 6 and 18 digits long. One way of thinking of the *sctId* is as a 64-bit integer, although it has an internal structure. Part of the structure is a *name-space* identifier, which is a 7-digit number that may be issued by SNOMED International to add unique local *extensions,* to support national, local or organizational needs. Extensions are not part of the content released internationally. All of the SNOMED CT codes shown in the Appendix are extensions.

Concepts

Concepts are clinical meanings that do not change. Every concept has a single identifier (*conceptId*). Concepts are organised into 19 top-level *hierarchies*. The international release of SNOMED CT has more than 350,000 concepts.

Descriptions

Descriptions are human readable labels for concepts in different languages and dialects. For example, American English and British English are different dialects. Every concept has a single fully specified name (FSN), a preferred term in each language and any number of synonyms. All descriptions are identified by a *descriptionId*. SNOMED CT defines more than a million descriptions.

Relationships

Relationships are used to link concepts together. Each relationship is defined using Object-Attribute-Value triples, where each part is a concept. Relationships can be used to define concepts, written using description logic (DL):

```
|concept|:|attribute|=|value|
```

For example, appendicitis has two parent relationships:

```
|appendicitis|:|IS A|=|disorder of appendix|
|appendicitis|:|IS A|=|inflammation of large intestine|
```

Appendicitis is both an appendix disorder and an inflammation of the large intestine. Appendicitis also has 15 child relationships which are specialisations of appendicitis.

SNOMED CT has more than 1.4 million relationships, identified by *relationshipId*.

Reference Terminology

SNOMED CT is a reference terminology, which means that concepts are defined in terms of their relationships with other concepts. The definitions are formal, machine-processable and support data aggregation and retrieval. This is a powerful idea, which solves many problems, but brings a good deal of complexity, which constrains maintenance and development. For example, every new concept added must be precisely placed in the correct hierarchy and ideally should be defined in terms of relationships with other concepts, although in practice much of SNOMED CT is not yet fully defined.

Value sets

In most practical applications only a tiny proportion of all concepts are applicable, so application designers specify sets of codes, called value sets, that may be used. Value sets are widely used in both applications and interoperability.

Computer-Based

SNOMED CT has never been published in any other way than as a set of computer files. It is designed for use with computers.

References

1. Benson T, Grieve G. Principles of health interoperability FHIR HL7 and SNOMED CT. 4th ed. London: Springer; 2021.
2. Standard computer dictionary: a compilation of IEEE standard computer glossaries. New York, NY: Institute of Electrical and Electronics Engineers; 1990.
3. Shannon C. A mathematical theory of communication. Bell Syst Tech J. 1946;27(379–423):623–56.
4. ISO/IEC. Guide 2: standardization and related activities—General vocabulary. Geneva: ISO 2004, definition 3.2.
5. Ayaz M, Pasha M, Alzahrani M, Budiarto R, Stiawan D. The fast health interoperability resources (FHIR) standard: systematic literature review of implementations, applications, challenges and opportunities. JMIR Med Inform. 2021;9(7):e21929.
6. Fielding RT. Architectural styles and the design of network-based software architectures. Irvine: University of California; 2000.
7. Sayeed R, Gottlieb D, Mandl KD. SMART markers: collecting patient-generated health data as a standardized property of health information technology. NPJ Digital Med. 2020;3(1):1–8.
8. Auerbach A, Bates D. Introduction: improvement and measurement in the era of electronic medical records. Ann Int Med. 2020;172(11_Supplement):S69-S72.
9. Bodenreider O, Cornet R, Vreeman D. Recent developments in clinical terminologies—SNOMED CT, LOINC and RxNorm. IMIA Yearbook of Med Inf. 2018;27(01):129–39.
10. McDonald C, et al (eds). Logical observation identifiers names and codes (LOINC) users' guide. Indianapolis, IN: Regenstrief Institute; 2017.
11. SNOMED CT Starter Guide. London: SNOMED International; 2017.
12. SNOMED CT Extensions: practical guide. V1.1 International Heath Terminology Standards Development Organisation 2021. http://snomed.org/extpg

Value of Health and Lives

Death Rates

During the twentieth century, average life expectancy rose consistently in almost all countries. Death rates for white American men and women aged between 45 and 54 fell by over 70% from over 1,400 per 100,000 in 1900 to under 400 in 2000, but since 2000 they rose by about 10%. The recent trend change in the USA is mainly due to what Case and Deaton call *deaths of despair* among white people without further education, caused by drugs, suicide and alcohol [1]. Deaths of despair have increased further since the COVID pandemic.

In England, mortality rates in the most deprived communities and the time spent in poor health have also increased during the decade 2010–2020 [2].

Death rates are one of the few measures where we have long time series, going back over 200 years, but they are a lagging indicator. We can do nothing for those who have died. Death is a simple binary indicator—you are either alive or dead.

In economic evaluation, we need to relate the benefits of an intervention to its costs. This implies placing a monetary value on reducing morbidity and avoiding deaths. There are two ways to do this. The first is to seek real-life examples of what people do to achieve this. This is the basis of the value of a statistical life (VSL) approach. The second is to ask people, as members of the general population, to say what they think they would do. This approach, referred to as preference judgements, is used in valuing quality in quality-adjusted life-years (QALY).

Value of a Statistical Life (VSL)

The value of a statistical life (VSL) is widely used by governments when considering safety and other policy initiatives. VSL is based on real-world data about how much people are willing to pay for a small reduction in their risks of death from traffic accidents, industrial injuries or adverse health conditions caused by environmental pollution. The US government's Environmental Protection Agency (EPA) explains the concept as follows:

> Suppose each person in a sample of 100,000 people were asked how much he or she would be willing to pay for a reduction in their individual risk of dying of 1 in 100,000, or 0.001%, over the next year. This reduction in risk would mean that we would expect one fewer death among the sample of 100,000 people over the next year on average. This is sometimes described as "one statistical life saved". Now suppose that the average response to this hypothetical question was $100. Then the total dollar amount that the group would be willing to pay to save one statistical life in a year would be $100 per person × 100,000 people, or $10 million. This is what is meant by the "value of a statistical life" [3].

Other ways of calculating VSL are to examine how much more people are paid in higher risk jobs, how much people will spend on buy safer but more expensive products, awards made by the courts, or simply asking people. All give broadly similar answers. These studies show that VSL is related to age by an inverse-U pattern, starting low, peaking between 40 and 50 years old and then gradually reducing [4].

The VSL approach has been used to assess and justify the costs and benefits of government policies such as the response to COVID-19 [5].

Preference Measures

Health preference research aims to provide quantitative estimates of the relative desirability of different options to different people in different places. People can be patients, the public, clinicians, suppliers, buyers, or regulators, but different groups value different things. For example, patients may seek improved subjective well-being, while doctors may aim to maximise what they can measure using blood tests.

Most people fear future physical disability more than mental illness. However, patients living with these health conditions adapt much more easily to disabilities than to mental health and they rate mental illness as worse than disability.

Preference research is used in two main ways.

1. First, to identify the dimensions or constructs that matter to different people. This is widely accepted as a good thing.
2. Secondly to generate numeric scores for each dimension or item, to allow a composite score or value to be created. This is more controversial.

Several different preference methods are available [6].

- Matching methods, where people provide numbers that will make them indifferent to the outcomes being valued. Examples are standard gamble (SG), time trade-off (TTO) and contingent variation.

- Choice-based methods, where people score the importance of attributes in a pairwise manner, such as discrete choice experiments (DCE), potentially all pairwise rankings of all possible alternatives (PAPRIKA) and best–worst scaling.
- Rating methods, where people allocate scores to different attributes, such as the simple multi-attribute rating technique (SMART) and visual analogue scales (VAS).
- Ranking methods, such as ranking attributes in order of importance.
- Pairwise comparison methods, such as the analytical hierarchy process (AHP).

Unfortunately, these different methods generate different results [7], which may be due to the noise and bias involved (see Chap. 5). Furthermore, most methods do not account of developments in behavioural economics, such as prospect theory, where gains and losses are not symmetrical. People regret losing $1,000 more than they value gaining $1,000 [8].

QALY Model

The QALY (Quality-Adjusted Life-Year) model is based on preference judgements and focuses on life expectancy. It has been a foundation for health economic evaluation for almost 40 years [7, 9]. In contrast, VSL focuses on deaths.

Some organisations, notably the National Institute for Clinical and Care Excellence (NICE) in the UK, require that health effects of interventions, especially new medicines, are expressed as changes in QALYs for cost-effectiveness analysis [10].

The QALY model combines mortality and morbidity into a single number using various levels of quality of life to represent morbidity. It takes account of both the quantity and quality of life by placing a value on time spent in different health states. Health status, expressed in terms of weighted life expectancy (QALY), is the sum across all health states of the time spent in each state multiplied by the relative value of that state, on a scale where *healthy* (or full health) has $qaly = 1$ and *dead* has $qaly = 0$.

For an individual i

$$\text{qaly}_i = \sum h_j t_j \tag{8.1}$$

where

j Indexes the states of illness including the states healthy and dead

h_j Utility score or weight attributed to state j, where $h_{healthy} = 1.0$ and $h_{dead} = 0$

t_j Expected duration of stay in state j

Σ Sum across all values of j.

This equation simplifies to length of life if only states of *alive* and *dead* are considered. Because $h_{dead} = 0$, there is no need to estimate the length of time spent in the state dead t_{dead}. The model allows for states worse than *dead*, which have negative values of h_j.

The basic QALY model can be extended for populations and to discount future health. Although, intuitively attractive and simple, QALYs remain controversial. They have been criticised on the grounds that they are not really utilities, do not encapsulate all relevant attributes and may not reflect social values [7].

Any good theory or model should predict what usually happens in practice, but the QALY model often predicts results that differ considerably from those expected. For example, the QALY model places a lower value on saving the life of a person who is more ill than the life of someone who is less ill, but most people are concerned to help those who have worst health and greatest need [11]. Also QALYs also value long life expectancies and capacity to benefit more than people say they do [12]. Unlike VSL, for example, QALYs value saving the life of a person aged 20 without dependents more than that of someone aged 40 with a family.

Empirical evidence about people's priorities at the end of life shows multiple differing views [13]. Writing as a surgeon, Rawles suggests that clinical focus is on the relief of suffering and prolonging life, but QALYs can lead to anomalies that he regards as absurd [14].

An EU-funded study tested the validity of some of the assumptions that underlie the scaling methods used in QALYs. QALY theory suggests that all people should prefer to live ten years in a wheelchair followed by death rather than five years, but a significant minority (28%) say they would not [16]. The authors suggest that the QALY theory fails to account for personal differences about medical outcomes. Many people would rather have a quick peaceful death rather than a drawn out demise with low quality of life.

There is not a consensus about to the basic assumptions built into the QALY model, such as linearity with quality and length of life, the effect of prognosis and number of dependents [15].

The arguments for and against QALYs are well documented [7, 9, 17], but few robust alternatives have emerged to combine morbidity and mortality into a single number [18]. Remedial approaches have focused on improving the classification schemes for describing patient states of illness, the methods used to obtain scales of valuations for different states and using QALYs in situations where the anomalies are less apparent, such as comparing treatments for the same conditions.

One alternative to QALYs are Disability-adjusted life years (DALYs), which are years of healthy life lost (QALYs are years of healthy life lived) [19]. Another approach is based on capabilities [20]. The capability approach uses a scale from 0 to 1 where 0 represents no capability and 1 represents 100% capability [21]. However, QALYs, DALYs and capability-based models are all variants of the same conceptual model. Each multiplies the number of years by the quality of those years.

At all levels, decision-makers are called upon to make trade-offs between programmes that aim to improve quality of life and those that aim to reduce the probability of fatalities. They need a way to help them, which combines morbidity and mortality aspects for use in economic evaluation and other decision-making.

Load Model

The Load model, set out below, is a possible candidate. It uses a different conceptual model incorporating some aspects of VSL. This section is a slightly modified version of that originally published [22].

The Load model is based on the idea that the primary objective of health services is the prevention and relief of morbidity and mortality caused by illness. The term Load represents the perceived consequences of morbidity and mortality to an individual or population. These are usually negative.

The key concepts are:

1. The state of being well has *load* = 0
2. All time after death has *load* = 0.
3. The *load* (impact) of death is attributed to the death event in the period in which it occurs. Death events may be treated as equal or weighted according to the age or context of death (as in VSL).
4. States of illness have a load based on subjective preferences using the same scale as death events.
5. For a population, load is the sum of the load due to death and illness within that population over a specified period. It is expressed as a rate (*load/period*). The choice of period is typically one year.

The basic equation for a population is:

$$\text{load} = mD + \sum l_j p_j \qquad (8.2)$$

where:

m Mortality rate expressed as the proportion of individuals dying during the period

D Load attributed to death events (assuming all deaths are considered equal)

j Indexes possible health states $1, 2 \ldots k$. The set of states includes the state healthy and the state dead

p_j The probability that an individual, who is alive at the start of the year, will be in state j at any time during the period. This is estimated point prevalence of state j ($p_j = N_j/N$) where N_j is the number of cases in state j and N is the population. For the population the sum of probabilities is 1, ($\sum p_j = 1$)

l_j The load attributed to being in state j for the period

Σ Sum over all values of j

The mortality component alone is mD, which reduces to mortality rate m if D is given an arbitrary fixed *load* of 1 ($D = 1.0$).

Similarly, the second expression reduces to point prevalence of illness if only one state j is considered, and l_j is given an arbitrary weight of 1 (excluding l_{well} and l_{dead}, which both have *load* = 0).

Other features can also be incorporated although they add to complexity. For example, expressions can be created to allow for different weights for D depending on the age and circumstances of death.

A special case of Eq. (8.2) is for one individual over one period. The period may be one or more years, survival following diagnosis or treatment, or remaining lifetime. For the remaining lifetime this gives:

$$\text{load}_i = \frac{D + \sum l_j t_j}{T} \qquad (8.3)$$

where:
D load attributed to death of individual i
l_j load attributed to being in state j for time unit (e.g. one year)
t_j number of time units (e.g. years) spent by individual i in state j
T remaining lifetime
Σ Sum over all values of j

To avoid dividing by zero, immediate death is allocated to the period in which it occurs.

A Worked Example

A worked example demonstrates the differences between the QALY and Load models using the single lifetime special case. This has been chosen because it is relatively easy to visualise for oneself. It is set out in six steps:

1. Preference estimation.
2. Derivation of value using QALY model for one year for illness state h
3. Derivation of value using Load model for one year for illness state l
4. QALYs for a hypothetical life
5. Load for a hypothetical life
6. Comparison of four alternative outcomes.

A Worked Example

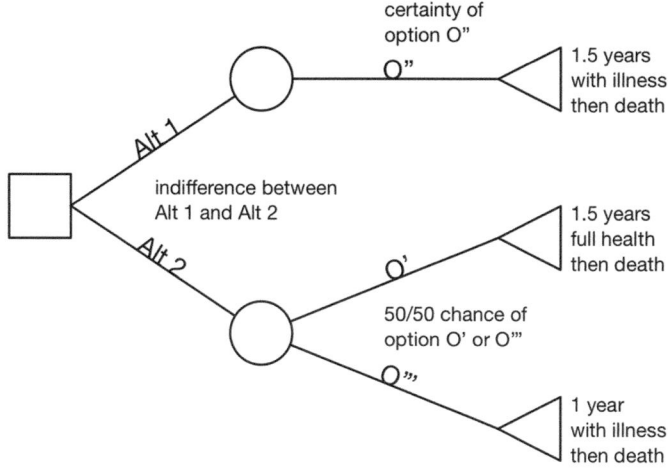

Fig. 8.1 Standard gamble (SG) example

(1) Preference estimation

Any method of preference estimation can be used, although some are easier to use than others. Possible methods include SG, TTO, DCE, VAS mapping and others [8, 23]. Here we use the standard gamble (SG), mainly because it is the most widely taught method of utility estimation although, in practice, it is one of the hardest to use [24]. See Fig. 8.1.

> A hypothetical judge, accepting the axioms of utility theory, expresses indifference to the following choice:
> EITHER (Alt 1) life expectancy of 1.5*years* with illness ($j = 2$) throughout (*outcome* O'')—this is the certainty option
> OR (Alt 2) a lottery with 50/50 chance ($p = 0.5$) of:
> EITHER 1.5*years* life expectancy with full health ($j = 1$) throughout (*outcome* O')—this is the best option
> OR 1.0*year* life expectancy with illness ($j = 2$) throughout (*outcome* O''')—this is the worst option

Where *outcome* O' is preferred to O'' which is preferred to O'''. In this example, 1.5 years of full health is preferred to 1.5 years with illness, which is preferred to 1 year of illness, each followed by death.

The indifference between certainty O'' and the lottery can be expressed in general terms as:

$$weight(O'') = p \times weight(O') + (1-p) \times weight(O''') \qquad (8.4)$$

where *weight*(O) is the utility attributed to outcome O.

(2) Derivation of qaly

Using the results of the standard gamble above

h_1 is good health ($h_1 = 1$), h_2 is illness (what we want to calculate) and h_3 is dead ($h_3 = 0$)

t_1 is time in best option ($t_1 = 1.5$), t_2 is time in certain option ($t_2 = 1.5$) and t_3 is time in worst option ($t_3 = 1.0$)

p is probability of best option ($p = 0.5$)

Using Eqs. (8.1) and (8.4), we obtain (leaving out the terms for $h_3 = 0$):

$$(h_2 \times t_2) = (h_1 \times t_1 \times p) + (h_2 \times t_3 \times (1-p))$$

$$(h_2 \times 1.5) = (1 \times 1.5 \times 0.5) + (h_2 \times 1 \times (1-0.5))$$

Multiply both sides by 2

$$3h_2 = 1.5 + h_2$$

$$h_2 = 0.75 \text{ for illness}$$

For reference, using the EQ-5D-5L five-level value set for England [25], this valuation ($h_2 = 0.75$) is consistent with EQ-5D-5L state 21,322 ($h = 0.751$)

> slight problems in walking about, no problems washing and dressing himself, moderate problems in doing usual activities (e.g. work, study, housework, family or leisure activities), slight pain or discomfort and slightly anxious or depressed.

(3) Derivation of load

Using a similar approach, we also calculate load l_2, where:

l_1 is good health ($l_1 = 0$), l_2 is illness (what we want to calculate) and l_3 is died during the year ($l_3 = 0$); D is value attributed to death ($D = -100$)

t_1 is time in best option ($t_1 = 1.5$), t_2 is time in certain option ($t_2 = 1.5$), t_3 is time in worst option ($t_3 = 1.0$)

T is total period until death ($T_1 = 1.5$, $T_2 = 1.5$, $T_3 = 1.0$)

p is probability of best option ($p = 0.5$).

Then using Eqs. (8.3) and (8.4), we get (leaving out the terms for $l_1 = 0$):

$$\frac{D + (l_2 \times t_2)}{T_2} = \left(\frac{D}{T_1} \times p\right) + \left(\frac{D + (l_2 \times t_3)}{T_3} \times (1-p)\right)$$

$$\frac{-100+(l_2 \times 1.5)}{1.5} = \left(\frac{-100}{1.5} \times 0.5\right) + \left(\left(\frac{-100+(l_2 \times 1)}{1.0}\right) \times (1-0.5)\right)$$

Multiply both sides by 3

$$3l_2 - 200 = 1.5\ l_2 - 250$$

$$1.5l_2 = -50$$

$$l_2 = -33.3$$

This may look complicated, but when broken down into its components, it is easier than it looks.

The results so far are summarised in Table 8.1, showing the main differences between the QALY and Load models.

(4) QALYs for a hypothetical life

Now we apply these values to a hypothetical life span for an individual from birth T_0 to his death. He is in full health for period $t_1 = 72$ years, falls ill (with constant severity) for period $t_2 = 3$ years and dies at the age of 75 $(t_1 + t_2)$.

His quality-adjusted life expectancy is given by Eq. (8.1):

$$qaly = \sum h_j t_j$$

This gives:

$$qaly = (1 \times 72) + (0.75 \times 3) = 74.25$$

In this example, the reduction due to morbidity is $75 - 74.25 = 0.75\,qaly$. The length of life (mortality) and morbidity components are 75 and 0.75 respectively (ratio of 100:1).

Table 8.1 Comparison of weights for the QALY and Load models for different states but the same judgement

	QALY model	Load model
Healthy (one year)	1.0	0
Illness (one year)	0.75	−33.3
Death (event)	0	−100
Dead (state)	0	0

(5) Load for a hypothetical life

Using the same inputs, *load* is given by Eq. (8.3) and simplifies as follows:

$$load = \frac{D + t_2 l_2}{t_1 + t_2}$$

where $D = -100$ and $l_2 = -33.3$:

$$load = \frac{-100 + (3 \times -33.3)}{75} = -2.67$$

In this example, the *load* due to mortality and morbidity are equal (−1.335 per year each).

The scales used to measure QALYs and Load are different. QALYs are a sum which should be maximised, but Load is a rate which should be as close to zero as possible.

The relative proportion of morbidity for QALY is 1% and for Load is 50%. A big difference!

(6) Surgery outcomes

In practice, we may want to examine the differences in outcomes when making important decisions. For example, our individual, aged 72, needs to decide whether to have a high-risk operation with three possible outcomes:

1. Do nothing. The prognosis is to live with symptoms for another 3 years, then die.
2. Operate unsuccessfully and die at the time of the operation.
3. Operate successfully and live without symptoms for another 10 years before dying suddenly of another cause.

This is not the type of decision that anyone would like to make, and it is oversimplified to make it easier to understand, but people make similar decisions every day in cancer surgery, for example.

We show the results in Table 8.2, based on the same judgement used earlier. Both *qaly* and *load* are calculated from age 72.

Table 8.2 Comparing four outcomes starting at age 72

Outcome	Qaly	Load
1. No operation. Illness is not relieved, dies age 75	2.25	− 66.7
2. Operation. Dies during operation, age 72	0	− 100
3. Operation. Illness is completely relieved, dies at 82	10	− 10

We can now calculate, using Eq. (8.4) above, the probability (p) of perioperative death for which this person would be indifferent between no treatment and having the operation for both QALY and Load models.

QALY model:

$2.25 = 0 + ((1-p) \times 10)$, so death during surgery is $p = 0.775$ and probability of success is $p = 0.225$.

Load model:

$-66.7 = (p \times -100) + ((1-p) \times -10)$, so death during surgery is $p = 0.63$ and probability of success is $p = 0.37$.

In this example, our hypothetical patient would be indifferent about having the operation, which has a 22.5% chance of success (the alternative being death during surgery) using the QALY model or 37% chance of success using the Load model. Again, a big difference (QALY is 64.4% more optimistic).

Discussion

Reduction of suffering (what we call *load*), rather than maximisation of health, was the focus of seminal papers by authors such as Culyer, Lavers and Williams [26], and Rosser and Watts [27], before Williams and Rosser both espoused QALYs [28]. Rosser and Watts used the QALY model using data from the General Household Survey to estimate the weighted life expectancy for the population of Great Britain [29]. They found that the morbidity component was small (1–3% depending on various assumptions) and suggested that complete elimination of all morbidity would have about the same effect as an overall increase in life expectancy of about one year. These results are similar to those in our QALY example. Given that life expectancy improved by about two years per decade throughout the twentieth century this result looks odd.

The original motivation for developing the Load model and describing it here is that the Load model produces results that appear to correspond a lot better with peoples' behaviour than does the QALY model. The QALY model has been widely accepted in health economics but a desire to understand anomalies is one of the reasons why new paradigms are developed [30].

References

1. Case A, Deaton A. Deaths of despair and the future of capitalism. Princeton University Press;2020.
2. Marmot M. Health equity in England: the Marmot review 10 years on. BMJ. 2020; 368: m693.
3. Environmental protection agency. Mortality risk valuation. https://www.epa.gov/environmental-economics/mortality-risk-valuation. Accessed 26 Oct 2021.
4. Viscusi WK. Pricing lives: guideposts for a safer society. Princeton University Press;2018.
5. Robinson L, Sullivan R, Shogren J. Do the benefits of COVID-19 policies exceed the costs? Exploring uncertainties in the age-VSL relationship. Risk Anal. 2021;41(5):761–70.

6. Marsh K, van Til JA, Molsen E, et al. Health preference research in Europe: a review of its use in marketing authorization, reimbursement, and pricing decisions—report of the ISPOR stated preference research special interest group. Value in Health. 2020;23(7):831–41.
7. Brazier J, Ratcliffe J, Salomon JA, Tsuchiya A. Measuring and valuing health benefits for economic evaluation, 2nd ed. Oxford University Press;2017.
8. Kahneman D, Tversky A. Prospect theory: an analysis of decision under risk. Econometrica. 1979;47(2):263–91.
9. Drummond MF, Sculpher MJ, Claxton K, et al. Methods for the economic evaluation of health care programmes, 4th ed. Oxford University Press;2015.
10. Timmins N, Rawlings M, Appleby J. A terrible beauty: a short history of NICE, the National Institute for Health and Care Excellence. Nonthaburi: Health Intervention and Technology Assessment Program (HITAP) 2016.
11. Schlander M. Measures of efficiency in healthcare: QALMS about QALYs? Z Evid Fortbild Qual Gesundhwes. 2010;104(3):214–26.
12. McHugh N, Baker RM, Mason H, et al. Extending life for people with a terminal illness: a moral right and an expensive death? Exploring societal perspectives. BMC Med Ethics. 2015;16(1):1.
13. Nord E. Cost-value analysis in health care: making sense out of QALYs. Cambridge University Press;1999.
14. Rawles J. Castigating QALYs. J Med Ethics. 1989;15:143–7.
15. Dolan P, Shaw R, Tsuchiya A, Williams A. QALY maximisation and people's preferences: a methodological review of the literature. Health Econ. 2005;14(2):197–208.
16. Beresniak A, Medina Lara A, Auray JP, et al. Validation of the underlying assumptions of the quality-adjusted life-years outcome: results from the ECHOUTCOME European project. Pharmacoeconomics. 2015;33(1):61–9.
17. Schlander M, Garattini S, Holm S, et al. Incremental cost per quality-adjusted life year gained? The need for alternative methods to evaluate medical interventions for ultra-rare disorders. J Comp Eff Res. 2014;3(4):399–422.
18. Reed JF. Moving the QALY forward or just stuck in traffic? Value in Health. 2009;12(suppl):S38-39.
19. Arnesen T, Nord E. The value of DALY life: problems with ethics and validity of disability adjusted life years. BMJ. 1999;319(7222):1423–5.
20. Sen A. Capability and well-being. In: Nussbaum M, Sen A, editors. The quality of life. Oxford University Press;1993. p. 270–293.
21. Coast J, Flynn TN, Natarjan L, et al. Valuing the ICECAP capability index for older people. Soc Sci Med. 2008;67:874–82.
22. Benson T. The Load model: an alternative to QALY. J Health Econ. 2017;20(2):107–13.
23. Torrance GW. Measurement of health state utilities for economic appraisal: a review. J Health Econ. 1986;5(1):1–30.
24. Gafni A. The standard gamble method: what is being measured and how it is interpreted. Health Serv Res. 1994;29(2):207–24.
25. Devlin N, Shah K, Feng Y, et al. Valuing health-related quality of life: an EQ-5D-5L value set for England. Health Econ. 2018;27(1):7–22.
26. Culyer AJ, Lavers RJ, Williams A. Social indicators: health. Social Trends. 1971;2:31–42.
27. Rosser R, Watts V. The measurement of hospital output. Int J Epidemiol. 1972;1:361–8.
28. Williams A. Discovering the QALY, or how Rachel Rosser changed my life. In: Oliver A, editor. Personal histories in health research. London: Nuffield Trust; 2005. p. 191–206.
29. Rosser R, Watts V. The measurement of illness. J Oper Res Soc. 1978;29(6):529–40.
30. Kuhn T. The structure of scientific revolutions. University of Chicago Press; 1962.

Part II
Measures

Patient-Reported Measures

Core Outcome Sets

Increasingly, the need has been recognised for groups of measures, or core outcome sets (COS), that work well together. Examples of programs that have been set up to create outcome sets are the Core Outcome Measures in Effectiveness Trials (COMET) initiative to assess effectiveness in trials and the International Consortium for Health Outcomes Measurement (ICHOM) to assess value in health care. Difficulties faced include the complexity of outcomes measurement, the large number of similar but siloed initiatives and lack of incentives from key influencers in the current healthcare environment [1].

The measures described in this, and subsequent chapters, measure different things that impact peoples' health and quality of life. Most measures are only moderately or weakly correlated [2].

Common properties of PROMs and PREMs have been introduced in Part I of this book. They include specialty-independence, brevity, ease of use, low reading age, a common format, data collection, reporting and data visualisation methods. These measures are used in tailoring care, quality improvement, service evaluation, clinical trials and as key performance indicators.

Taxonomy

A taxonomy is simply an organising framework for things. When the number of things rises above a certain number it is useful to organise them into a framework that helps people find what they want. Often, but not always, a taxonomy is organised as a hierarchy, where each node is a sub-class of its parent and a parent to its children.

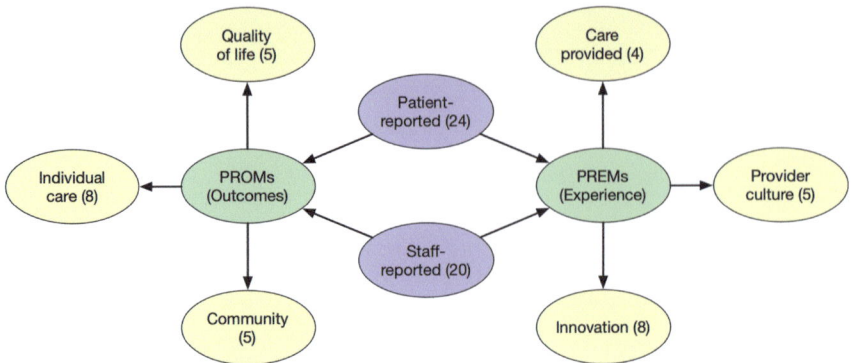

Fig. 9.1 Top levels of the taxonomy

Biological taxonomy, pioneered by Carl Linnaeus in the eighteenth century, is a well-known example, where all of life is classified hierarchically into kingdom, phylum, class, order, family, genus, and species.

In a similar way, this book is organised into parts, chapters and sections and sub-sections within chapters. In general, there is no right or wrong way to do this, just so long as it is useful.

In the area of PROMs and PREMs, we could organise a taxonomy based on many different principles, such as type of respondent, type of measure, domain covered, diagnostic group, method of administration and so on. We use the first three of these as shown in Fig. 9.1, which shows the top three levels of the structure we have developed.

The numbers in parentheses show the number of different measures in each group. Measures are not counted twice if they are identical, or almost identical, for both patient and staff responses. The colours represent different levels of the hierarchy.

The taxonomy shown here is closely based on that previously published [3], updated with more recent developments. The measures, their items and options are shown in Table 9.1 for patient-reported measures. Staff-reported measures are discussed later in Chap. 17.

Patient and Staff-Reported

Patient-reported and staff-reported measures cover the same domains, but sometimes there are important differences between them in terms of content and mode of administration. It helps to consider these roles separately.

Patients are subjects of care, but proxies, such as family members, may respond on behalf of patients. Patients have unique perception of their own perceptions about how they feel and their personal experience of healthcare.

Staff, including clinicians, admin staff and volunteers, provide care within an organisational structure. Staff see many patients and the data collection process is usually simpler. Many staff-reported measures (Chap. 17) have been adapted from patient-reported measures.

At the next level, the two broad categories of measure are person-reported outcome measures (PROMs) and person-reported experience measures (PREMs).

PROMs Domains

PROMs refer to the impact on individuals as perceived by the rater. They include measures of: Quality of life, Individual care, and Community.

Quality of life measures include people's health status, personal wellbeing, fatigue and sleep patterns. These are usually about patients, recorded by patients themselves or proxies on their behalf.

Individual care measures include health confidence, shared decision-making, self-care, behaviour change, adherence to treatment (eg, medication) and acceptance of loss. Individual care is typically based on interactions between patient and clinician (staff); both groups have their own perception of the outcome, which may differ.

Community measures include external and environmental factors such as social determinants of health, loneliness, neighbour relationships and personal safety. This is mainly related to how and where people live and so are usually best answered by patients.

PREMs Domains

PREMs measure people's perception of the service provided. These include measures of Care provided, Provider culture, and Innovation.

Care provided covers both individual services and the way that services work together. Both patients and staff have views about the quality of care provided.

Provider culture measures aspects of each health and care organisation's policies and practice. Staff have much more direct knowledge and experience of their organisation's culture than do patients.

Innovation focuses on the impact of specific innovations, such as digital health applications and new ways of working. Staff are invariably involved and patients less frequently.

Option Sets

The following option sets are used:

- None—Extreme (None, A little, Quite a lot, Extreme)
- Strongly agree—Strongly Disagree (Strongly agree, Agree, Neutral, Disagree)

- Excellent—Poor (Excellent, Good, Fair, Poor)
- Strongly agree—Strongly disagree (Strongly agree, Agree, Disagree, Strongly disagree)
- Hardly ever—Always (Hardly ever, Occasionally, Sometimes, Always)

Each option set has four response options, scored 3, 2, 1 and 0 respectively. The best option (the ceiling) has the highest score and can be thought of as being as good as it gets. Because this is the desired outcome, it does not result in a troubling ceiling effect, whereby the measure is unable to detect valuable improvements. In some cases, such as when asking about symptoms where Disagree is the best option, the scoring scheme needs to be reversed. A floor effect (the worst option) is more problematic, because things can always get worse. In general, if a respondent is at the floor, this calls for remedial action. Intermediate options can be regarded as being less good than the ceiling and less bad than the floor, respectively. A summary score is calculated as the sum of the four items (where a measure has four items). Mean scores for a population are calculated with a maximum score of 100 (ceiling) and a minimum score of 0 (floor) for both items and summary scores.

Table

Details of each measure are shown in Table 9.1 for patient-reported measures. This is set out with three columns:

1. Name: a short easy to understand name or label. The name is usually positively worded, but not always. For example, the health status (howRu) measure has an item for pain or discomfort. Here, the best (highest) score comes from having no pain. The English language is better at describing some aspects negatively.
2. Text used in survey: text as presented to the respondent. In practice each survey also contains a preamble. This is not shown here, because it is usually context-specific and contains locally specific instructions and context. Where the text includes terms in square brackets, these can be replaced by a more appropriate phrase, such as a project or product name.
3. Options: the response options measure how much the respondent currently perceives something to be a problem. Many measures ask about agreement with positively worded statements using a scale from strongly agree to disagree. This column also contains a pointer to the chapter (if applicable) where the measure is discussed in more detail.

We have also developed measures for use staff (Chap. 17) and by unpaid carers or caregivers (see Chap. 18). These share many of the same features.

Quality of Life

Quality of life is what patients want. Quality of life measures include people's health status, personal wellbeing, fatigue and sleep patterns. These are about patients, recorded by patients themselves or proxies on their behalf.

Health Status
Health status (howRu) is sometimes referred to as health-related quality of life (HRQoL). This was the first in the family [4]. (See also Chap. 11).

Personal Wellbeing
Personal Wellbeing Score (PWS) is based on the Office of National Statistics ONS4. Unlike ONS4 all items are worded positively, and it has a summary score [5]. (See also Chap. 12).

Person-Specific Outcome
The individualised person specific outcome measure gives staff an opportunity to list two issues that they would like to be addressed [6]. (See also Chap. 14).

Sleep
Sleep hygiene is an important determinant of health and wellbeing [7].

Fatigue
Fatigue is a common presenting complaint in primary care and can have a large impact on quality of life [8].

Individual Care

Measures of individual care include health confidence, shared decision-making, self-care, behaviour change, adherence to treatment (e.g. medication) and acceptance of loss. Individual care is typically based on interactions between patient and clinician (staff); both groups have their own perception of the outcome, which may differ.

Health Confidence
Health confidence (HCS) covers people's confidence about looking after their own health [9]. (See also Chap. 13).

Self-Care
Self-care includes self-management of diet, physical activity, weight and medication [10].

Shared Decisions
Shared decisions (SDM) covers patients' involvement in clinical decisions, including their understanding of the choices and the risks and benefits of each [11]. (See also Chap. 13).

Behaviour Change
Behaviour change covers capability, opportunity and motivation (conscious and unconscious) to change behaviour based on Michie's COM-B model [12]. (See Chaps. 4 and 16).

Adherence
Adherence includes remembering to take medications and treatment, and to follow instructions as specified, given side-effects or recovery [13].

Acceptance of Loss
Acceptance of loss covers how people cope with loss, learn to live with events including recognition of capabilities and change, how to do things differently and to move on with life, along the lines of the grief cycle [14].

Community
Community measures include external and environmental factors such as social determinants of health, social contact, loneliness, neighbour relationships and personal safety. This is mainly related to how and where people live.

Social Determinants
Social determinants of health impact health and care outcomes but are outside the clinical system. Education, autonomy, housing and poverty all play a major role in determining peoples' health outcomes [15]. (See also Chap. 15).

Social Contact
Social contact is an important determinant of health and wellbeing. This measure focuses on peoples' perception of their social relationships in a positive way [16]. (See also Chap. 15).

Loneliness
This measure is included as an alternative to social contact (above), based on guidance from the Office of National Statistics (ONS) [17]. (See also Chap. 15).

Neighbour Relationships
Neighbour relationships, community cohesion and social capital are impacted by how well people know, trust and help each other [18].

Personal Safety
Personal safety covers physical safety (e.g. from injury) and emotionally safety (from verbal abuse or discrimination), which may occur either inside your own home or when you go out [19].

Care Provided

Care provided covers both individual services and the way that services work together. Patients and staff have views about the quality of care provided.

Patient Experience
Patient experience (howRwe) covers peoples' perception of the care and service provided by a specific service in terms of compassion, communication, access and organisation [20]. (See also Chap. 10).

Service Integration
Service integration captures how well services collaborate [21]. (See also Chap. 11).

Provider Culture

Provider culture measures aspects of each health and care organisation's policies and practice. Staff usually have better direct knowledge and experience of the culture than patients (See also Chap. 17).

Privacy
Privacy covers patients' perceptions of data protection, sharing and information governance [22].

Innovation

Innovation focuses on the impact of specific innovations, such as digital health applications and new ways of working. Staff are invariably involved and patients less frequently. (See also Chap. 16).

Digital Confidence
Digital confidence assesses people's confidence in using digital apps and similar devices [23].

Product Confidence
Product confidence covers understanding of and confidence in using a specific innovation, application or product [24].

User Satisfaction
User satisfaction focuses on people's perception of how much an innovation is useful and easy to use, availability of help and overall satisfaction [25].

Digital Readiness
Digital readiness covers how ready people are to use digital innovations and their innovativeness [26].

Training
The Training measure is based on Kirkpatrick's four levels: Reaction, Learning, Behaviour and Results [27].

Table 9.1 Patient-reported Measures

Name	Text used in survey	Options
Quality of life		
Health status	*How are you today? (Past 24 h)*	None—Extreme
Pain/discomfort	Pain or discomfort	Chapter 11
Distress	Feeling low or worried	
Disability	Limited in what you can do	
Dependence	Require help from others	
Personal wellbeing	*How are you feeling in general?*	Strongly agree—Disagree
Life satisfaction	I am satisfied with my life	Chapter 12
Worthwhile	What I do in my life is worthwhile	
Happy	I was happy yesterday	
Not anxious	I was NOT anxious yesterday	
Person specific outcome	*List one or two issues you would like help with*	None—Extreme
Issue 1	Issue 1 [write in]	Chapter 14
Issue 2	Issue 2 [write in]	
Sleep	*Thinking about your recent sleep pattern*	Strongly agree—Disagree
Sleep at same time	I go to sleep at the same time	
Wake at same time	I wake up at the same time	
Wake refreshed	I wake up feeling refreshed	
Sleep well	I sleep well	
Fatigue	*Thinking about getting tired*	Strongly agree—Disagree
Energy level	I usually have enough energy	
Tire quickly	I don't tire too quickly	
Able to concentrate	I can usually concentrate well	
Stamina	I can keep going if I need to	

(continued)

Table 9.1 (continued)

Name	Text used in survey	Options
Individual care		
Health confidence	*How do you feel about caring for your health?*	Strongly agree—Disagree
Knowledge	I know enough about my health	Chapter 13
Self-management	I can look after my health	
Access to help	I can get the right help if I need it	
Shared decisions	I am involved in decisions about me	
Self–care	*How well do you look after yourself?*	Strongly agree—Disagree
Diet management	I manage my diet well	
Exercise management	I manage my physical activity well	
Weight management	I manage my weight well	
Meds management	I manage my medication well	
Shared decisions	*Thinking about [your plan]*	Strongly agree—Disagree
Know benefits	I know the possible benefits	Chapter 13
Know downside	I know the possible downside	
Know choices	I know that I have choices	
Fully involved	I feel fully involved	
Behaviour change	*Thinking about [this behaviour]*	Strongly agree—Disagree
Capability	I am able to do it (skills and tools)	Chapter 4
Opportunity	Nothing prevents me from doing it	
Conscious motive	I choose to do it	
Automatic motive	I do it without thinking	
Adherence	*Do you follow treatment instructions?*	Strongly agree—Disagree
Remember	I remember to do it	
Go on if I feel bad	I don't stop if I feel bad	
Go on if I feel better	I don't stop if I feel better	
Treatment satisfaction	I am happy with my treatment	
Acceptance of loss	*Have you learnt to live with what's happened?*	Strongly agree—Disagree
New capability	I know what I can and cannot do	
Recognize loss	I see how my life has changed	
Change activity	I do things differently now	
Move on	I have moved on	
Community		
Social determinants	*Thinking about how you live*	Strongly agree—disagree
Education	I have had a good education	

(continued)

Table 9.1 (continued)

Name	Text used in survey	Options
Self-efficacy	I feel in control of what I do	Chapter 15
Housing	I am happy about where I live	
Poverty	I have enough money to cope	
Social contact	*Thinking about your friends and family*	Strongly agree—Disagree
People to talk to	I have people to talk to	Chapter 15
People to confide in	I have someone I can confide in	
People to help	I have people who will help me	
Do things with others	I do things with others	
Loneliness	*How often do you*	Hardly ever–Always
No one to talk to	Have no one to talk to?	Chapter 15
Feel left out	Feel left out?	
Feel alone	Feel alone?	
Feel lonely	Feel lonely?	
Neighbour relationships	*Thinking about your neighbours*	Strongly agree—Disagree
Know each other	We know each other	
Trust each other	We trust each other	
Share information	We share information	
Help each other	We help each other	
Personal safety	*Thinking about your personal safety*	Strongly agree—Disagree
Safe at home	I feel safe at home	
Respected at home	I feel respected at home	
Safe outside	I feel safe outside home	
Respected outside	I feel respected outside home	
Care provided		
Patient experience	*How are we doing?*	Excellent—Poor
Kindness	Treat you kindly	Chapter 10
Listen/explain	Listen and explain	
Prompt	See you promptly	
Organised	Well organised	
Service integration	*How well do services work together?*	Strongly agree—Disagree
Services talk together	Services talk to each other	Chapter 10
Service knowledge	Staff know what other services do	
Repeat story	I don't have to repeat my story	
Services work together	Different services work well together	
Provider culture		
Privacy	*Thinking about how we use your data*	Strongly agree—Disagree

(continued)

Table 9.1 (continued)

Name	Text used in survey	Options
Data is safe	My data is kept safe and secure	
Data shared as needed	My data is only shared as needed	
Can see/check data	I can see and check my data	
Happy about data use	I am happy about how my data is used	
Innovation		
Digital confidence	Digital devices include computers, mobiles & tablets	Strongly agree—Disagree
Digital usage	I use a digital device frequently	Chapter 16
Peer usage	Most of my friends use digital devices	
Access to help	I can usually get help if I am stuck	
Confident digitally	I feel confident using most digital devices	
Product confidence	How do you feel about [this product]?	Strongly agree—Disagree
Frequent user	I use it frequently	Chapter 16
Confident user	I feel confident using it	
Know benefits	I know the potential benefits	
Know problems	I know potential problems	
User satisfaction	What do you think of [this product]?	Strongly agree—Disagree
Helps me	It helps me do what I want	Chapter 16
Easy to use	It is easy to use	
Can get help	I can get help if I need it	
Product satisfaction	I am satisfied with this product	
Digital readiness	New ideas in this field of work	Strongly agree—Disagree
Digital use	I use a digital device frequently	Chapter 16
Confidence	I feel confident using most digital devices	
New ideas needed	New ideas are needed	
Keep up to date	I keep up with new ideas	
Training	Thinking about this course	Strongly agree—Disagree
Reaction	It was relevant and I enjoyed it	Chapter 16
Learning	I have learnt new things	
Behaviour	I shall use what I have learnt	
Results	The impact should be good	

References

1. Moloney R, Messner D, Tunis S. The increasing complexity of the core outcomes landscape. J Clin Epidemiol. 2019;116:150–4.
2. Black N, Varaganum M, Hutchings A. Relationship between patient reported experience (PREMs) and patient reported outcomes (PROMs) in elective surgery. BMJ Qual Saf. 2014;23(7):534–42.
3. Benson T. Measure what we want: a taxonomy of short generic person-reported outcome and experience measures (PROMs and PREMs). BMJ Open Quality 2020; 9: e000789.
4. Benson T, Whatling J, Arikan S, McDonald D, Ingram D. Evaluation of a new short generic measure of HRQoL: howRu. Inform Prim Care. 2010;18:89–101.
5. Benson T, Sladen J, Liles A, et al. Personal Wellbeing Score (PWS)—a short version of ONS4: development and validation in social prescribing. BMJ Open Qual. 2019; 8:e000394.
6. Benson T. Person-specific outcome measure (PSO) for use in primary and community care. BMJ Open Quality 2021; 10:e001379.
7. Walker M. Why we sleep. London: Allen Lane; 2017.
8. Sharpe M, Wilks D. Fatigue. Br Med J. 2002;325:480–3.
9. Benson T, Potts HWW, Bark P, et al. Development and initial testing of a Health Confidence Score (HCS). BMJ Open Qual. 2019;8:e000411.
10. Shrivastava SR, Shrivastava PS, Ramasamy J. Role of self-care in management of diabetes mellitus. J Diabetes Metab Disord. 2013;12(1):14.
11. Barry MJ, Edgman-Levitan S. Shared decision making—the pinnacle of patient-centered care. N Engl J Med. 2012;366(9):780–1.
12. Michie S, Van Stralen MM, West R. The behaviour change wheel: a new method for characterising and designing behaviour change interventions. Implement Sci. 2011;6(1):42.
13. Lam WY, Fresco P. Medication adherence measures: an overview. BioMed Res Int 2018; 2015:217047.
14. Kübler-Ross E. On death and dying. New York: Simon & Schuster; 1969.
15. Marmot M. The health gap: the challenge of an unequal world. Lancet. 2015;386:2442–4.
16. Goodman A. Measuring your impact on loneliness in later life. London: Campaign to end loneliness; 2015.
17. Snape D, Martin G. Measuring loneliness—guidance for use of the national indicators on surveys. Office for National Statistics; 2018.
18. Putnam RD. Bowling alone: the collapse and revival of American community. New York: Simon and Schuster; 2001.
19. Bilsky W. Fear of crime, personal safety and well-being: a common frame of reference. Universitäts-und Landesbibliothek Münster; 2017.
20. Benson T, Potts HWW. A short generic patient experience questionnaire: howRwe development and validation. BMC Health Serv Res. 2014;14:499.
21. The NHS Long Term Plan. London: NHS 2019. www.longtermplan.nhs.uk
22. van Staa T-P, Goldacre B, Buchan I, et al. Big health data: the need to earn public trust. Br Med J.
23. Prensky M. Digital natives, digital immigrants. On the Horizon. 2001;9(5):1–6.
24. Pappas N. Marketing strategies, perceived risks, and consumer trust in online buying behaviour. J Retail Consum Serv. 2016;29:92–103.
25. Stoyanov S, Hides L, Kavanagh D, et al. Mobile app rating scale: a new tool for assessing the quality of health mobile apps. JMIR Mhealth Uhealth. 2015; 3(1):e27.
26. Rogers EM. Diffusion of innovations. 5th ed. The Free Press; 2003.
27. Kirkpatrick DL, Kirkpatrick JD. Evaluating training programs: the four levels. 3rd ed. San Francisco CA: Berrett-Koehler; 2006.

Patient Experience 10

Background

Health care is a service and all patients should have a good experience of care. Patient experience is a key measure that can be used to improve quality, governance, accountability and choice [1]. However, it is a complex, multi-attribute concept that reflects patients' individual experiences of receiving care.

A short definition is that patient experience is *the sum of all interactions, shaped by an organization's culture, that influence patient perceptions across the continuum of care*. This makes it clear that patient experience is about patient perceptions, relating to interactions across the continuum of care and it is shaped by the organization's culture and processes. Many other definitions of patient experience have also been put forward [2].

Patient experience measures are PREMs and are about the healthcare provider that has provided that experience. In this respect PREMs differ from PROMs, which are all about the subject of care.

Traditional patient experience surveys have been criticised for survey length, infrequent sampling frequency, slow feedback and failure to use results to improve care and quality [3, 4]. Many are long. The English General Practice Patient Survey, which was described in Chap. 4, is almost 3,000 words long with 61 questions.

The Hospital Consumer Assessment of Healthcare Providers and Systems (HCAHPS—pronounced H-caps) survey about hospital stays in the US has 29 questions and 1,070 words. HCAHPS covers care from nurses and doctors, the hospital, post-discharge and questions about the patients' mode of admission, general and mental health, education, ethnicity, race and language spoken at home.

Patient experience focuses on different aspects explicitly, in contrast to patient satisfaction, which is more of an assessment. Some people are satisfied with standards of care that others find inadequate. Patient experience is usually more objective than patient satisfaction.

Development

Most patient experience measures are specific to particular settings, such as inpatient stays, general practice appointments, outpatient visits, maternity care, care homes or home care. A generic measure would allow comparisons between different settings along the patient pathway.

In developing a patient experience measure, we identified a need for a short generic instrument to capture patients' perceptions of the service they had experienced with minimal effort, that could give rapid feedback to all stakeholders in a way that was comparable, scalable, and economical.

Devising Items

The development and validation of any new measure is not something to be undertaken lightly. It often takes much longer than expected, even after recognising that this is not a quick job.

The first stage includes setting the scope, sourcing, and refining the items. This is a key stage because if the items are not right, nothing else can be. Each step may need to be repeated numerous times, sometimes over several years.

Scope

The first step is to agree the project scope. At a minimum, the scope statement should clearly state why action is needed, set the project boundaries and specify SMART objectives (SMART objectives have been described in Chap. 4).

The case for action should be a concise, compelling and comprehensive statement of why a new measure is needed. It describes the context, problem, and user needs. It should also set out the consequences of doing nothing.

Scope delineation shows the project boundary—what is in and out of scope. Part of this step is to agree upon the approach to be used. Some measures focus on a particular event, others on a longer time interval.

Any attempt to re-use existing deliverables in ways that are outside their original scope needs a strong health warning.

Sourcing Items

The next step is sourcing potential items. Many measures are commissioned by someone with a clear idea of what they want. It is tempting for the designer to simply give them what they ask for. However, the commissioner is only one (important) source of ideas and does not answer the questions.

Questionnaires are completed by patients. It is always a good idea to find out what matters most to them and to understand their first-hand experience of living with their conditions. This can be done through formal or informal focus groups.

Published papers are another useful source. Most papers go through a lengthy period of review and revision and represent well-baked opinions. They show what other people have done and identify alternative theories and conceptual frameworks that can influence thinking. Qualitative research can be helpful, especially when combined with expert opinion from experienced researchers and clinicians.

Prototype questionnaires need to be tested. Pay close attention to free text comments and items that are not answered.

Refining the Items

Substantial effort is often needed to refine items to mean just what you want them to mean to the reader. It is hard to get this exactly right. Measure content can evolve over several years and hundreds of iterations.

It is often a challenge to find just the right short generic phrase that applies across the whole continuum of care. For example, clinical staff are often referred to using role-specific terms such as GP, dentist, surgeon, nurse or paramedic. One option is to use a term such as "clinician" but this term is not widely used outside healthcare and many patients may not understand it. The English language may have up to a million words, but the average person uses no more than 20,000. It is better to avoid using words that many people may not use or know.

In patient experience we quickly identified four key dimensions that we wanted to cover:

1. **Compassion.** This includes how you are treated as a person including compassion, empathy, emotional support, politeness, dignity, respect, and privacy. The final text was *Treat me kindly*.
2. **Communication.** This broad area includes all aspects of two-way communication between patient and clinician. It includes patient engagement, information provision, education, choice, consent, shared decision-making (SDM), and empowerment. The final text was *Listen and explain*.
3. **Timeliness.** This covers all types of delay, waiting, access, cancellation and responsiveness; it includes the delay between referral and appointment, waiting in the clinic to be seen and the time taken to respond to a call bell. The final text was *See me promptly*.
4. **Reliability.** This covers how well patients perceive the unit to be managed, including safety, dependability, efficiency and whether information such as lab results are available when and where needed and acted upon appropriately. The final text was *Well organized*.

The four final items only have 11 words in total yet cover a very wide spectrum of concepts. In some cases, less is more. For more information, see the original paper [5].

Options

The strength of each item is rated using four options: *Excellent, Good, Fair* and *Poor*. Each option is also indicated in four mutually supporting ways to reduce cognitive effort, avoid the need for training and to improve face validity. These are written labels, colour (green, yellow orange and red), position decreasing in

Patient experience

How are we doing? (our recent care)

	Excellent	Good	Fair	Poor
Treat you kindly	🙂	🙂	😐	☹
Listen and explain	🙂	🙂	😐	☹
See you promptly	🙂	🙂	😐	☹
Well organised	🙂	🙂	😐	☹

Fig. 10.1 The howRwe patient experience measure

excellence from left to right, and smiley face emojis. Note that colour, position and emojis are optional. You cannot use them if the questionnaire is completed during a telephone call.

In addition to the items and options, each measure usually includes an overarching preamble statement. In this case it is *How are we doing? (our recent care)*. The text in parentheses can be changed to fit local contexts.

The final form, showing the preamble, items and options is shown in Fig. 10.1.

Many PROMs and PREMs specify a recall period, such as *over the past month…* However, human memory is far from perfect. Most people cannot remember what they had for dinner a couple of days ago unless it was a special meal.

Memory is also susceptible to bias. For example, in a blinded randomized control study of memories of colonoscopy, the difference between the two arms of the experiment was that in first group the scope remained inserted for up to three minutes longer at the end of the procedure than for the second. Those who had the longer procedure perceived it to be significantly less unpleasant than those who had the shorter procedure, and they were more likely to have a repeat procedure if required [6].

Scoring

For analysis and reporting at the individual level, each item is given a score on a 0–3 scale as follows: Excellent = 3; Good = 2; Fair = 1 and Poor = 0.

A summary or aggregate score, the Patient Experience or howRwe score is calculated by adding the individual scores for each item, giving a scale with 13 possible values from 0 (4 × *Poor*) to 12 (4 × *Excellent*).

When reporting the results for a group (comprising more than one respondent), the mean scores are transformed arithmetically to a 0–100 scale, where 100 (the

Development

Table 10.1 Length and readability. (Source [5])

Instrument	No. of items	No of Words	FKG Readability Grade	Reading age
howRwe patient experience	4	29	2.2	7.2
NHS Friends & Family Test	1	44	6.6	11.6
GS-PEQ	10	150	8.8	13.8
EUROPEP 2006	23	214	8.1	13.1
PPE-15	15	467	7.1	12.1
NHS Adult Inpatient Survey 2013	76	3,353	7.3	12.3
GP Patient Survey 2014	62	2,922	6.8	11.8

ceiling) indicates that all respondents rated *Excellent* and 0 (the floor) that all respondents rated *Poor*. This is done by multiplying individual scores by 100 and dividing by 3 for items and by 12 for summary scores. This allows item scores to be compared with summary scores on the same scale.

Readability

Respondent burden depends on brevity and readability. Brevity is easy to measure—just count the words. Readability is more nuanced.

Table 10.1 shows the word count and Flesch Kincaid Grade (FKG) and reading age statistics for several patient experience measures (NHS FFT [7], GS-PEQ [8], EUROPEP 2006 [9], Picker PPE-15 [10], NHS Adult Inpatient Survey 2013 [11] and the GP Patient Survey 2014 [12]. These figures are based on the full published text, including instructions, framing statements, items and options. Readability is discussed in more detail in Chap. 3.

The howRwe patient experience measure has a much lower FKG score, and hence reading age, than any of the other measures. These are broadly comparable in readability, but not in word count.

Case Study

The data used in this case study comes from the pre-operative assessment clinic at the Nuffield Orthopaedic Hospital, Oxford before and after changes were introduced. These were designed to make the clinic run more smoothly and reduce delays for the benefit of both patients and staff [5].

Data was collected from May 2013 to February 2014. Changes were made to the appointment scheduling system and the physical layout of the clinic at the end of August 2013. Data was collected using an iPad towards the end of their visit, which typically lasted several hours. The purpose of the visit was to help patients prepare for their operation, discharge and recovery. Patients would usually see several different staff members during this visit, such as the surgeon, anaesthetist, phlebotomist, physiotherapist, occupational therapist, nurses and clinic staff. No identifiable information was collected (data was anonymous) and patients freely consented to complete the task.

This study had two main objectives:

- to assess the impact of the changes made.
- to assess the performance of the howRwe patient experience measure including the frequency distribution and validity.

Distribution

Patients were asked to complete the survey by a clinic receptionist who tended not to do this when the clinic was very busy. It was not practical to measure the number of people who declined to complete the survey.

Tables 10.2 and 10.3 summarise the frequency distribution and descriptive statistics for all data (before and after changes) and for all items and the howRwe summary score. The distributions are skewed towards excellent. This known as a ceiling effect. A ceiling effect is when a large proportion of responses are at the best possible category; a floor effect is when they are at the worst possible category.

Here, a ceiling effect is no bad thing because excellence is what we want. A floor effect would not be good, because things can always get worse. Here, 68% of all item responses were Excellent, 26% Good, 5% Fair and 1% Poor. 48.8% of all respondents chose Excellent for all four items.

The frequency distribution shows items where improvement may be needed. Only 1.0% and 2.0% respectively rated *Treat me kindly* and *Listen and explain* as less than good, but this was 13.1% and 7.9% respectively for *See me promptly* and *Well organised*.

Table 10.2 also shows the mean individual level score and using the 0–100 scale their mean, 95% confidence intervals and standard deviations for each item and the howRwe summary score.

Internal Structure
Each item in a measure or test should measure different aspects of the same construct. This implies that they should be moderately correlated, but neither too much nor too little.

Case Study

Table 10.2 Distribution and descriptive statistics for each item and the howRwe summary score

Item	Treat me kindly	Listen and explain	See me promptly	Well organized	howRwe summary score
Responses (n)	828	828	828	828	828
Excellent	671 (81.0%)	609 (73.6%)	447 (54.0%)	530 (64.0%)	–
Good	148 (17.9%)	202 (24.4%)	273 (33.0%)	233 (28.1%)	–
Fair	7 (0.8%)	16 (1.9%)	90 (10.9%)	51 (6.2%)	–
Poor	2 (0.2%)	1 (0.1%)	18 (2.2%)	14 (1.7%)	–
Mean score (raw)	2.80	2.72	2.39	2.54	10.44
Mean score (0–100)	93.2	90.5	79.6	84.8	87.0
95% CI	92.3–94.2	89.3–91.6	77.9–81.3	83.3–88.1	85.9–88.1
Standard Deviation	14.7	16.7	25.5	22.9	16.4

Table 10.3 Distribution of howRwe summary scores (n = 828)

Score	0	1	2	3	4	5	6	7	8	9	10	11	12
n	1	0	0	1	5	8	21	25	123	56	77	107	404
%	0.1	–	–	0.1	0.6	1.0	2.5	3.0	14.9	6.8	9.3	12.9	48.8

The internal structure of the howRwe patient experience measure was explored by examining the correlations between each pair of items, as shown in Table 10.4. The correlations all lie in the desired range 0.39–0.71, which are moderate to strong.

Exploratory factor analysis of the items found a single factor explaining 67% of the variance, demonstrating one-dimensionality as required.

The internal coefficient of reliability (Cronbach's α) was satisfactory ($\alpha = 0.82$; 95% CI: 0.79–0.83). It is generally recommended that Cronbach's α be in the range 0.7–0.9. This indicates that it is appropriate to use an overall summary score as well as the individual item scores [13].

Validation

Validity testing involves collecting the arguments for and against the use of results from a measure in a specific context. This is most easily done by testing hypotheses such as:

Table 10.4 Intra-item correlation matrix (95% CI) (n=828)

	Treat me kindly	Listen & explain	See me promptly	Well organized
Treat me kindly	–	0.71 (0.67–0.74)	0.39 (0.33–0.44)	0.51 (0.46–0.56)
Listen & explain		–	0.47 (0.42–0.52)	0.56 (0.51–0.60)
See me promptly			–	0.70 (0.66–0.73)
Well organized				–

1. Administrative items (promptness and organization) improved significantly after the new appointment scheduling system was introduced and the physical layout was changed.
2. Clinical items (compassion and communication) were not changed significantly.
3. Patient experience was associated with patient satisfaction as measured by the NHS Friends and Family Test (FFT) [7]. The FFT is discussed later in this chapter.
4. Patient experience (as measured by howRwe) was not associated with patients' health status. Health status was measured by howRu [14]. HowRu is discussed in Chap. 11.

Before and After

The first objective of this project was to test whether scores improved after making some changes to the way that the clinic was organized. Table 10.5 shows the mean before and after scores and the mean change (after − before) with 95% confidence intervals (CI), for each item. Also shown are the results of t-tests and Mann–Whitney U tests and the probability (p) that these come from the same population. The criterion is $p < 0.05$.

It can be seen that there is little difference in the clinical aspects (*Treat me kindly* and *Listen and explain*), which are very good both before and after the changes. However, there is a big improvement in the administrative aspects (*See me promptly* and *Well organized*) after the changes, which demonstrates that, as perceived by patients, the changes have been for the better.

Both parametric and non-parametric statistical tests (t-test and Mann–Whitney test) show similar results and confirm that there is a statistically significant change in the administrative items but not in the clinical items. The howRwe patient experience summary score also significantly improves, but not as much as for *See me promptly* and *Well organized*.

Table 10.5 Item and howRwe summary scores before and after changes to the clinic systems. This also shows confidence intervals (CI), t-test and Mann–Whitney test results with p values

Item	N	Treat me kindly	Listen and explain	See me promptly	Well organized	howRwe summary score
Before score	278	93.9	89.4	71.5	78.9	83.4
95% CI		92.1–95.6	87.5–91.4	68.5–74.5	76.2–81.6	81.3–85.5
After score	550	92.9	91.0	83.7	87.8	88.9
95% CI		91.7–94.1	89.6–92.4	81.6–85.8	85.9–89.7	86.9–90.9
Mean change (After–Before)		−1.0	+1.6	+12.2	+8.9	+5.5
95% CI		−1.4 to −0.6	1.1–2.0	11.6–12.9	8.4–9.5	4.6–6.2
t-test (t)		−0.91	1.24	6.69	5.38	4.55
p (t-test)		0.37	0.22	<0.001	<0.001	<0.001
Mann–Whitney U		74,516	79,025	94,126	89,342	91,196
p (M-W)		0.38	0.30	<0.001	<0.001	<0.001

Other Measures

The questionnaire also included the NHS Friends and Family Test (FFT) (see below).

We also recorded each person's health status using the howRu measure [14]. The correlation between the howRwe patient experience score and howRu was $r = 0.02$ (CI − 0.04–0.09), indicating that the two measures are independent, as hypothesised.

Taken together these findings support the validity of the howRwe patient experience measure in this study.

Service Integration

When people living with multiple conditions are asked about their healthcare, many say that they would like to see better integration between different services. They dislike having to repeat their stories time and again; they don't think different services share information well between them and think that some staff do not know what other services do. Above all, they would like healthcare services to work as if they are one joined-up service, not a set of independent fiefdoms.

Service integration is one of the core premises of patient-centered care but conflicts with the traditional medical model. The governance structure of medicine favours the development of specialty-specific silos. From early in their careers doctors are encouraged to specialise in specific conditions and modes of treatment, which creates barriers to integration.

The traditional focus of patient experience measures has been on a single service to the patients seen by it, not integration across different services. This problem is of little importance if a patient only has one condition, which can be treated by a single specialist. However, most money is spent on people living with multiple conditions.

Figure 10.2 shows the Service Integration measure developed because of these considerations. The four items relate to:

- how well services communicate—*services talk to each other*
- patients' perceptions of staff awareness of what other services do—*staff know what other services do*
- whether patients need to repeat their stories endlessly—*I don't have to repeat my story*
- how well different services collaborate as a team—*different services work well together*

The preamble is *how well do services work together?* The options are *Strongly agree*, *Agree*, *Neutral* and *Disagree*.

The scores obtained are often quite poor, which shows that this issue is of real concern to patients.

Service integration

How well do services work together?

	Strongly agree	Agree	Neutral	Disagree
Services talk to each other	😀	🙂	😐	☹️
Staff know what other services do	😀	🙂	😐	☹️
I don't have to repeat my story	😀	🙂	😐	☹️
Different services work well together	😀	🙂	😐	☹️

Fig. 10.2 Service Integration measure

Friends and Family Test

The NHS Friends and Family Test (FFT) was introduced across the NHS in England in 2013, for use by patients at every encounter [7]. It may be the biggest source of patient opinion in the world, with over 86 million responses (November 2021).

The original FFT had a single question (*How likely are you to recommend [this service] to friends or family if they needed similar care or treatment*) with a five-point scale from *Extremely likely* to *Extremely unlikely* plus a *don't know* option. It was inspired initially by the Net Promoter Score but with important differences in wording, options and analysis [15]. The original question received quite a lot of criticism [16]. It was modified in 2019 [17]. The following description relates to the revised version.

Changes included: the descriptive framework (question and options) were changed; it was no longer recommended that the FFT question be placed first in a longer questionnaire; the wording of the free-text question could be changed locally; the instructions relating to the timing requirements were relaxed, and no response rate data would be published centrally.

Several aspects did not change: the FFT should be asked of all patients; all responses are anonymous; providers can choose how to collect the data (e.g., pen and paper, SMS text, webpage, tablet); a free text question is required but providers can ask more than one if they wish; providers can add additional questions; data is submitted monthly; and providers can publish their own data locally, using for example, *you said, we did* formats.

The FFT descriptive framework has:

- Framing text, which may be tailored to the service. The wording is typically: *Thinking about [the service we provide]…*
- Mandatory standard question: *Overall, how was your experience of our service?*
- Response scale with six options: *Very good; Good: Neither good nor poor: Poor; Very poor; Don't know.*
- Free text question such as: *Please can you tell us why you gave your answer,* or: *Please tell us about anything we could have done better.* This is regarded as the most important part of the FFT.
- Optional tick box to indicate that the respondent is willing for their comments to be published. Any data that could identify patients should not be published.

Translations are available in 20 languages. Providers should use their own judgement about the best time to collect the FFT.

Each provider submits data monthly to a central repository, along with counts of the number of patients accessing services that month. For inpatients and day cases the site, ward and specialty are recorded.

FFT results are not comparable across organisations due to differences in data collection methods, timings, demographic characteristics and case mix. However, the results for a service can be used as time series to show improvement or a decline. Quantitative data may be used within the provider to monitor changes and by commissioners and regulators to assess patient engagement.

The free text data helps identify issues that can be resolved, to identify themes where improvement is possible and, alongside complaints and national survey results, to provide insight into what could be changed. The FFT guidance suggests that providers focus mainly on the free text feedback and what has been done with it, rather than response rates and scores [17].

As with all measures, what you get out of the FFT depends on the effort you devote to understanding the answers. The main value of FFT lies in the text comments. In general, people have to devote more effort to understand a set of text comments than to understand numerical results, such as the average score and distribution. Qualitative analysis of text comments can be rewarding but it needs a lot of commitment and skill to identify the key themes and to specify what can be changed to make things better.

References

1. Ahmed F, Burt J, Rowland M. Measuring patient experience: concepts and methods. Patient. 2014;7:235–41.
2. Wolf J, Neiderhauser V, Marshburn D, et al. Defining patient experience. Patient Exp J. 2014;1(1):7–19.
3. Coulter A, Locock L, Ziebland S, Calabrese J. Collecting data on patient experience is not enough: they must be used to improve care. BMJ. 2014; 348:g2225.
4. Robert G, Cornwell J. Rethinking policy approaches to measuring and improving patient experience. J Health Serv Policy. 2013;22:67–9.
5. Benson T, Potts HWW. A short generic patient experience questionnaire: howRwe development and validation. BMC Health Serv Res. 2014;14:499.
6. Redelmeier DA, Kahneman D. Patients' memories of painful medical treatments: real-time and retrospective evaluations of two minimally invasive procedures. Pain. 1996;66(1):3–8.
7. The friends and family test. London: NHS England 2014; Publications Gateway Ref No. 01787.
8. Sjetne I, Bjertnaes O, Olsen R, et al. The Generic Short Patient Experiences Questionnaire (GS-PEQ): identification of core items from a survey in Norway. BMC Health Serv Res. 2011;11:88.
9. Wensing M, Baker R, Vedsted P, et al. EUROPEP 2006 Revised Europe Instrument and User Manual. TOPAS Europe Association; 2006.
10. Jenkinson C, Coulter A, Bruster S. The Picker Patient Experience Questionnaire: development and validation using data from in-patient surveys in five countries. Int J Qual Health Care. 2002;14:353–8.
11. Picker Institute Europe: NHS adult inpatient survey 2013. Oxford; 2013.
12. Ipsos MORI. The GP patient survey. London: 2014.
13. Streiner DL, Norman GR, Cairney J. Health measurement scales: a practical guide to their development and use. 5th ed. Oxford University Press; 2015.
14. Benson T, Sizmur S, Whatling J, et al. Evaluation of a new short generic measure of health status: howRu. Inform Prim Care. 2010;18:89–101.

15. Robert G, Cornwell J, Black N. Friends and family test should no longer be mandatory. BMJ. 2018;360:1–2.
16. Reichheld F. The one number you need to grow. Harv Bus Rev. 2003;81(12):46–55.
17. Using the Friends and Family Test to improve patient experience. NHS England and NHS Improvement 2019; Guidance Reference: 000938. https://www.england.nhs.uk/wp-content/uploads/2019/09/using-the-fft-to-improve-patient-experience-guidance-v2.pdf.

Health Status   11

Background

This chapter covers health status; the next chapter covers personal wellbeing. Health status is sometimes also called health-related quality of life (HRQoL), while wellbeing is sometimes also referred to as happiness. We will not indulge in semantic niceties, but it is important to recognise that health status and wellbeing are different. Health status focuses mainly on functional capability, while wellbeing focuses on how people feel.

Health services need a way to measure the effectiveness of treatments that they get paid to deliver. The results that matter are those perceived by patients. The challenge is to measure the benefits in a practical way, which is applicable to all patients and care settings, and provides immediate, useful feedback to patients, clinicians and managers [1].

Routine health status measurement helps screen for problems, promotes patient-centred care, aids patients and doctors to take decisions, improves communication amongst multi-disciplinary teams and monitors progress of individuals or groups of patients and the quality of care in a population [2, 3]. These have been outlined in more detail in Chap. 1.

However, for various reasons, some of which have been described in Chaps. 4 and 5, routine use of health status measures in day-to-day clinical practice remains rare.

Two influential families of generic health status measures are SF-36 [4] and its derivatives such as SF-12, [5] and the EuroQoL EQ-5D [6].

These tools were designed for and are used widely in clinical research and population surveys. This chapter describes these instruments and the newer R-Outcomes *howRu* measure.

Two short case studies are provided. The first is a point-in-time study which compares *howRu* with SF-12. The second case study compares the generic EQ-5D-3L with the condition-specific Oxford Hip and Knee scores in a large sample of NHS patients before and after hip and knee replacement surgery. It shows the effect size (ES) of using different instruments to measure the same procedures.

SF-36 and SF-12

The Short-Form 36 (SF-36) questionnaire has 36 questions. It typically takes between five and fifteen minutes to complete, so it is not many peoples' idea of being short. However, it is short in comparison with the original 245-question Medical Outcome Survey, on which it is based [4]. In clinical trials, SF-36 is the most widely used health status measure and the original paper has more than 40,000 citations. It has been less widely used in routine clinical care.

SF-36 is a generic measure, applicable to a wide range of types and severities of health conditions, including multiple conditions. Generic measures compare the health status of patients with different conditions and with the general population. They address both physical and mental concepts and measure each concept in several ways.

Conceptually, SF-36 has eight sub-scales: physical functioning (PF); role limitations due to physical health problems (RP); bodily pain (BP); general mental health (MH); role limitations due to emotional problems (RE); vitality, energy or fatigue (VT) and general health perceptions (GH). One question, change in health status over the past year is not used in scoring. Most questions use a 4-week recall period.

A shorter version of SF-36 with 12 items (known as SF-12) is also used widely. It was designed to fit onto a single page and to be completed in less than two minutes. It has more than 15,000 citations [5].

Both SF-36 and SF-12 provide two main indicators, the physical component summary (PCS) and the mental component summary (MCS), reflecting mental and physical symptoms. PCS and MCS are based on normal distributions with a mean of 50 and standard deviation of 10; high is good. So, a PCS score of 40 is one standard deviation below the average.

Norm-based distributions are familiar in IQ scores, where the mean is 100 and the standard deviation is 15. For example, an IQ of more than 115 is more than one standard deviation above the average (about 1,590 in every 10,000 people). An IQ score of over 145 is three standard deviations above average; this is unusual (about 13 in every 10,000 people) but not extremely rare. It is 16,000 times more likely than winning the EuroMillions lottery jackpot with one ticket.

A generic preference-based measure of health (SF-6D) has been developed for use with both SF-36 and SF-12 data. This generates utility values which can be used in QALY calculations [6].

The overall structure of the SF-36 and SF-12 surveys, showing the components and sub-scales is shown in Fig. 11.1.

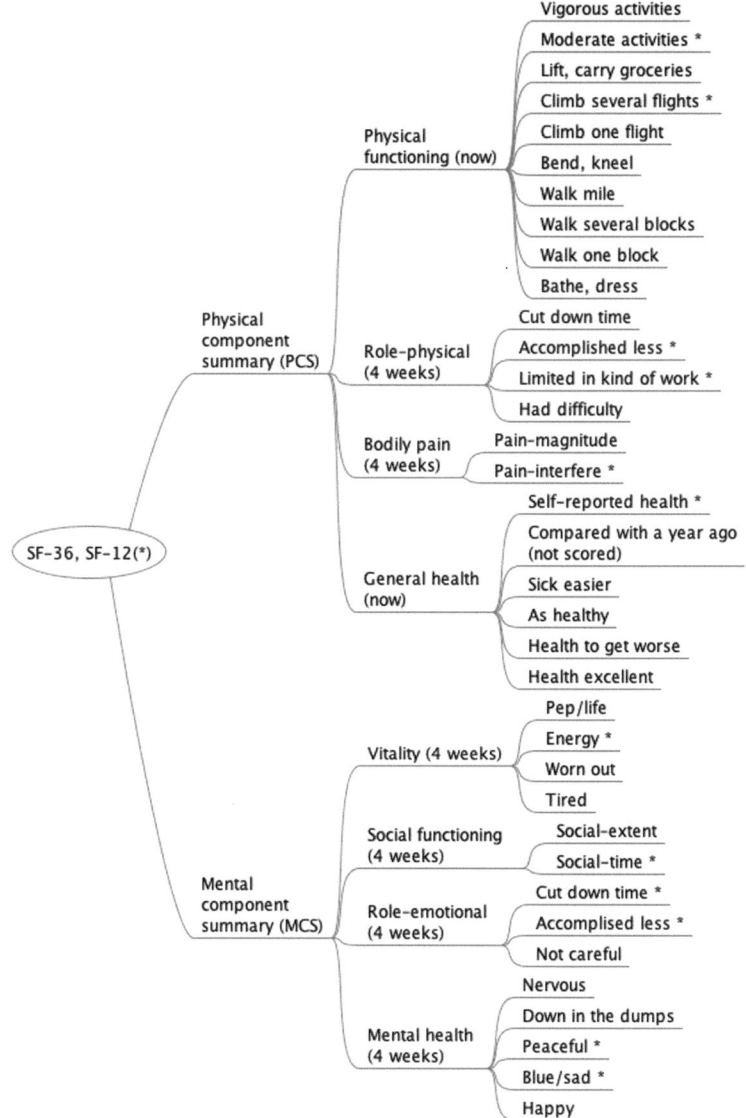

Fig. 11.1 Overall structure of SF-36 and SF-12. SF-12 items are marked by *. Recall periods are shown in parenthesis

EQ-5D

Another widely used generic measure is EQ-5D. The international EuroQoL group was founded in 1986 to develop the EQ-5D health status measure [7]. EQ-5D is a standardised generic self-completion measure of health status, for clinical use in and economic appraisal and population surveys, and to support the calculation of quality-adjusted life-years (QALYs) in cost-utility analysis.

EQ-5D has two main parts: the descriptive system plus its associated weighting system, and a visual analogue scale (EQ-VAS). First, we describe the EQ-5D-3L descriptive system, which has five dimensions (mobility, self-care, usual activities, pain/discomfort and anxiety/depression). Each dimension has three response options, typically (1) none/absent, (2) moderate/some and (3) unable/extreme, creating 243 (3^5) possible states.

For example, a patient with a migraine-like pain might report a score such as 11231 meaning:

1—I have no problems in walking about
1—I have no problems with self-care
2—I have some problems with performing my usual activities
3—I have extreme pain or discomfort
1—I am not anxious or depressed.

A value set (also known as a tariff) is used to weight each possible health state, using a scale from 1 (best conceivable health state) through dead (value 0) to the worst conceivable health state (which usually has a negative value) [8]. The resulting score is known as the EQ-5D-3L Index (EQ-Index).

Many tariffs have been produced; the most widely used one is for the UK general population [9]. Weights are subtracted from a maximum value of 1.0 using values shown in Table 11.1. In addition, if one or more dimensions indicates either a moderate problem (score 2) or an extreme problem (score 3), then an additional constant of −0.081 is subtracted; if one or more dimensions is scored 3 an additional constant of −0.269 is subtracted.

The value for profile used in the example above (11231) is therefore 0.228 made up from: 1.0 minus 0.081 (*any score of 2 or more*), minus 0.269 (*any score of 3*), minus 0.036 (*usual activity 2*), minus 0.386 (*pain/discomfort 3*).

Table 11.1 EQ-5D weights subtracted from 1.0 (UK tariff, 1997) [9]

Item score	Any	Mobility	Self-care	Usual activity	Pain/Discomfort	Anxiety/Depression
1. (No problem)	0	0	0	0	0	0
2. (Moderate problem)	−0.081	−0.069	−0.104	−0.036	−0.123	−0.071
3. (Extreme problem)	−0.269	−0.314	−0.214	−0.094	−0.386	−0.236

When used in QALY calculations, this is interpreted as meaning that 4.39 years in this state is deemed to be equivalent to one year in good health (1 divided by 0.228).

The second part of the instrument, the EQ visual analogue scale (EQ-VAS), is a 20 cm vertical thermometer anchored at 0 (worst imaginable health state) and 100 (best imaginable health state). The patient marks their present state by drawing a line from a box marked *Your own health today* to the visual analogue scale. The VAS also provides an alternative way to calculate weights [8].

A revised version of EQ-5D with five levels (EQ-5D-5L) was published in 2011 [10]. This adds two new response levels: one between original Level 1 (no problems) and Level 2 (moderate/some problems), and another between the Level 2 and Level 3 (severe problems). In addition, the most severe response level for Mobility was changed from "confined to bed" to "unable to walk about". There were also some changes in the instructions for marking overall health today on the visual analogue scale (VAS).

A UK value set was published in 2018 [11]. Unfortunately it comes with caveats; EQ-5D-3L and EQ-5D-5L are not interchangeable, and this valuation study has not been endorsed by NICE. The differences between results using the 3L and 5L versions are large, usually a reduction in health gain, and the direction can be unpredictable [12]. The issue of generating preference values for health states is controversial, an issue which has been discussed in Chap. 8.

howRu Health Status Measure

Around 2006 the author recognised a need for a generic health status measure for routine use in clinics. It would need to be very short, quick to use and designed for electronic data collection. Conceptually, health status measures record patients' perceptions of how they feel and what they can do. The name of the instrument, *howRu*, stems from the first question that a clinician asks at a consultation, namely: "How are you?" For full details of the development, see the original paper [13].

The origins of *howRu*'s descriptive system can be traced back to the work of Rachel Rosser, who developed a classification with eight classes of disability and four classes of distress, which she used to measure hospital output in terms of differences between admission, discharge and follow-up [14].

howRu measures health in terms of how the patient is feeling, physically and mentally, and how much they can do, in terms of loss of function and independence. Our approach is that of assessment now, rather than recall. Assessment captures the presence, absence, severity or intensity of a concept, while recall is based on recollection and memory, which is less reliable [15].

The wording, design and scoring system of *howRu* evolved through more than 150 iterations, using pilot studies, feedback from colleagues and members of the public, desk research including literature review, dictionaries and thesauri. The purpose was to use simple, widely-understood terms and descriptions, in order to

Health Status

How are you today? (past 24 hours)

	None	A little	Quite a lot	Extreme
Pain or discomfort	🙂	😐	☹️	😖
Feeling low or worried	🙂	😐	☹️	😖
Limited in what you can do	🙂	😐	☹️	😖
Require help from others	🙂	😐	☹️	😖

Fig. 11.2 howRu health status measure

reduce the risk of ambiguity and to ensure that as many people as possible could use it reliably and consistently without training or support.

The descriptive system is illustrated in Fig. 11.2. It has four items:

- Discomfort—this is intended to cover the severity of physical symptoms including breathlessness, itch, dizziness and nausea. The item wording seen by the respondent is: *Pain or discomfort.*
- Distress—this relates to emotional symptoms such as anxiety, stress, fatigue and depression. The item wording is *Feeling low or worried.*
- Disability—includes work, home and leisure activities. The item wording is: *Limited in what you can do.*
- Dependence—covers lack of autonomy, self-care and other activities of daily living. The item wording is: *Require help from others.*

The severity of each item is rated using four levels: *None, A little, Quite a lot, Extreme*. These are indicated in mutually supporting ways to minimise cognitive load:

- Written labels: *None, A little, Quite a lot,* and *Extreme*. The wording used is deliberately slightly ambiguous. For example, *A little* for *Pain or discomfort* could refer to its intensity or its duration or both. We seek an overall perception of how much bother it is causing.
- Colour: green, yellow, orange and red. This is based on the familiar traffic light system.
- Position: increasing in severity from left to right.
- Smiley face emojis, which show smile, neutral, sad and miserable respectively.

The preamble is *How are you today? (past 24 h)*. The phrase *(past 24 hours)* indicates that today means the whole 24 hours not just right now, because many people experience symptoms at different times of the day.

The resulting matrix, with four items and four levels, provides 256 (4^4) different possible combinations.

For analysis and reporting, each level is allocated a score on a 0–3 ordinal scale, with: *Extreme* = 0, *Quite a lot* = 1, *A little* = 2, and *None* = 3.

The summary *howRu* score is calculated by adding the scores for each item, giving a range from the floor, 0 (4 × *Extreme*), to the ceiling, 12 (4 × *None*).

When reporting results for a cohort, both item scores and the summary score are transformed to a scale from 0 (all *Extreme*) to 100 (all *None*). A higher score indicates better health status.

Case Study 1

Method

This case study describes the properties of the *howRu* health status measure in a point-in-time study of 2,751 people living with long-term conditions and compares this with SF-12. This study used an early version of *howRu*, which had some minor differences from the current version described above. The current wording is used here because the changes do not alter the results in any important way. For details as used, see the original paper [13].

The data was collected using computer-assisted telephone interview with a standard script during Summer 2008 in two regions of the United Kingdom using a random-digit dialling procedure. All respondents were screened to establish that they had one or more of 21 common long-term conditions, ranging from asymptomatic high blood pressure to cancer. The survey collected data about gender, age group, and the duration of the principal condition. SF-12 data was collected before the *howRu* data. Incomplete records were removed, but all *howRu* data was complete.

Distribution of Scores

The results were checked for a broad distribution and floor effect (not possible to detect further deterioration). We were not concerned about a ceiling effect (patients report no symptoms) because that is what we want.

The frequency distribution for each *howRu* item is shown in Table 11.2.

The distribution of the howRu health status summary score is shown in Table 11.3. The range of response rates for each option ranged from 4.9% (extreme distress) to 58.4% (no dependence).

Tables 11.2 and 11.3 show that each item and the *howRu* health status summary score cover a broad spectrum of patients with long term conditions. The standard deviations are quite high, which is as expected for patients with a broad range of conditions. If all patients were similar we would expect smaller standard deviations.

Table 11.2 Distribution and descriptive statistics for each item and the howRu summary score

	Pain or discomfort	Feeling low or worried	Limited in what you can do	Require help from others	howRu summary score
None	1199 (43.6%)	1521 (55.3%)	1029 (37.4%)	1608 (58.4%)	–
Slight	626 (22.8%)	663 (24.1%)	695 (24.8%)	443 (16.1%)	–
Quite a lot	701 (25.5%)	431 (15.7%)	713 (25.9%)	500 (18.2%)	–
Extreme	225 (8.2%)	136 (4.9%)	314 (11.4%)	200 (7.3%)	–
Responses (n)	2751	2751	2751	2751	2751
Mean (raw)	2.02	2.30	1.89	2.26	8.46
Mean (0–100)	67.2	76.6	62.9	75.2	70.5
95% CI	66.0–68.5	75.5–77.7	61.6–64.2	74.0–76.5	69.5–71.5
St. Dev.	33.6	30.2	34.6	33.2	26.0

Table 11.3 Distribution of howRu summary scores (n = 2751)

Score	0	1	2	3	4	5	6	7	8	9	10	11	12
n	25	37	61	92	145	197	207	210	276	234	289	382	596
%	0.9	1.3	2.2	3.3	5.3	7.2	7.5	7.6	10.0	8.5	10.5	13.9	21.7

Internal Structure

The internal structure of *howRu* was explored by examining the correlations between each pair of items. Correlations between *howRu* items should be moderate but strongest amongst the three 'physical' items of *howRu* (*Pain or discomfort*, *Limited in what you can do* and *Require help from others*). The results confirm this (Table 11.4). All correlations were significant at the $p < 0.01$ level (2-tailed).

Cronbach's α was 0.80, which suggests that the *howRu* items measure different aspects of a single underlying continuum. Cronbach's α measures the extent to which items are consistent with each other and may be used together reliably as a single score. α increases with the number of items in a scale (*howRu* has only 4 items) and should be in the range 0.70 and 0.90, depending on the measurement purpose. An α of 0.80 is in the center of the desired range for a scale of this length and is suitable for individual-level measurement [16].

Case Study 1

Table 11.4 Intra-item correlation matrix between *howRu* items (n = 2751)

	Feeling low or worried	Limited in what you can do	Require help from others
Pain or discomfort	0.40	0.58	0.47
Feeling low or worried		0.45	0.39
Limited in what you can do			0.65

Table 11.5 Correlations between *howRu* items and PCS-12 and MCS-12 (n = 2751)

howRU item	PCS-12	MCS-12
Pain or discomfort	0.64	0.28
Feeling low or worried	0.33	0.59
Limited in what you can do	0.71	0.36
Require help from others	0.64	0.35
howRu summary score	0.74	0.49

Validity

The SF-12 Health Survey provided a criterion for assessing the validity of the *howRu* results.

The correlations between each *howRu* item (including the summary score) and the PCS-12 and MCS 12 scores are shown in Table 11.5.

As expected, the correlation between the three 'physical' items of *howRu* and the SF-12 Physical Components Summary (PCS-12) are stronger (0.64, 0.71 and 0.74) than with the SF-12 Mental Components Summary (MCS-12) (0.28, 0.36 and 0.35 respectively).

Similarly the correlation of the 'mental' item of the *howRu* (*feeling low or worried*) is stronger with MCS-12 ($r = 0.59$) than with PCS-12 ($r = 0.33$). All correlations are statistically significant.

The correlation between the *howRu* summary score and PCS-12 and MCS-12 scores are $r = 0.74$ and $r = 0.49$ respectively. The correlation of the *howRu* summary score and the sum of PCS-12 and MCS-12 are $r = 0.81$, which is very strong. This is strong evidence indicating that *howRu* and SF-12 measure the same things.

Case Study 2

One of the main uses of PROMs is to assess the cost-effectiveness of different healthcare interventions using methods of technology appraisal. One task is to calculate an incremental cost-effectiveness ratio (ICER). ICER is calculated by dividing the difference in the costs of two interventions by the differences in the effectiveness. In cost-utility analysis, effectiveness is usually measured in quality adjusted life years

(QALY). The ICER is often expressed in the form such as £20,000 per QALY. The strengths and weaknesses of the QALY are discussed in Chap. 8.

How effectiveness is measured is important. Since 2009, every patient receiving hip and knee replacement surgery in the English NHS has been asked to complete a PROMs questionnaire before and six months after surgery. This is one of the longest-running routine PROMs studies anywhere; anonymised datasets are published on the web for further analysis.

The information presented here uses the NHS PROMs provisional results (2019–2020), which were the latest available data at the time of writing [17]. For additional information, see the original paper, based on older data [18].

Data collected includes the Oxford Hip Score (OHS), [19] Oxford Knee Score (OKS) [20] and EQ-5D-3L Index (EQ-Index) and the EQ-5D-3L Visual Analogue Score (EQ-VAS) for both hips and knees [7]. The OHS and OKS are similar and were developed by the same team and have a close family resemblance. Both have 12 questions and use an aggregate scoring scheme. The OHS is shown in Table 11.6. EQ-5D-3L has been described above.

All of these instruments were developed as measures of benefit as perceived by patients, so we might expect the results for each measure to be comparable for both pre-op measures and changes. We might also expect scores and changes in scores to be highly correlated.

Unfortunately, each measure uses a different scale, making comparisons difficult. The range for each measure from floor (worst possible state) to ceiling (best possible state) are as follows: OHS and OKS 0 to 48, EQ Index −0.594 to 1.0, EQ-VAS 0 to 100. To simplify comparison, scores were transformed to 0–100 range using the floor and ceiling scores as anchors. If all respondents scored at the floor, the mean score would be 0; if all scored at the ceiling the mean score would be 100. For example to convert EQ-Index to 0–100 scale take the mean score, add 0.594, multiply by 100 and divide by 1.594.

Results

The key results using 0–100 scales are shown in Tables 11.7 and 11.8; these show the mean scores, standard deviation, number of respondents and percentage of missing values for each measure before (Pre-Op), 6 months later (Post-Op) and the change calculated as the difference between Post-Op and Pre-Op scores for hips and knees respectively

Across all measures, the outcome for hip replacement is better than the outcome for knees. The OHS and OKS are more sensitive to change than the EQ-Index (46.8 vs. 28.9 for hips and 36.1 vs. 21.4 for knees). EQ-Index is more sensitive than the EQ-VAS (28.9 vs. 14.1 for hips and 21.4 vs. 7.9 for knees).

Effect Size

The effect size (ES) of any intervention is defined as the average change divided by the baseline SD [21]. For hip replacement, ES of OHS is 2.74, for EQ-Index is 0.50,

Table 11.6 Oxford Hip Score showing questions and options. Very minor changes have been made from original for formatting reasons

Oxford Hip Score (OHS)	
During the past four weeks	
(1) How would you describe the pain you usually had from your hip?	1. None
	2. Very mild
	3. Mild
	4. Moderate
	5. Severe
(2) Have you had any trouble with washing and drying yourself (all over) because of your hip?	1. No trouble at all
	2. Very little trouble
	3. Moderate trouble
	4. Extreme difficulty
	5. Impossible to do
(3) Have you had any trouble getting in and out of a car or using public transport because of your hip? (whichever you tend to use)	1. No trouble at all
	2. Very little trouble
	3. Moderate trouble
	4. Extreme difficulty
	5. Impossible to do
(4) Have you been able to put on a pair of socks, stockings or tights?	1. Yes, easily
	2. With little difficulty
	3. Moderate difficulty
	4. Extreme difficulty
	5. No, impossible
(5) Could you do the household shopping on your own?	1. Yes, easily
	2. With little difficulty
	3. Moderate difficulty
	4. Extreme difficulty
	5. No, impossible
(6) Before the pain from your hip became severe? (with or without a stick)	1. No pain/>30 min
	2. 16–30 min
	3. 5–15 min
	4. Around the house
	5. Not at all
(7) Have you been able to climb a flight of stairs?	1. Yes, easily
	2. With little difficulty
	3. Moderate difficulty
	4. Extreme difficulty
	5. No, impossible

(continued)

Table 11.6 (continued)

Oxford Hip Score (OHS)	
During the past four weeks	
(8) After a meal (sat at a table), how painful has it been for you to stand up from a chair because of your hip?	1. Not at all painful
	2. Slightly painful
	3. Moderately painful
	4. Very painful
	5. Unbearable
(9) Have you been limping when walking, because of your hip?	1. Rarely/never
	2. Sometimes or at first
	3. Often, not just at first
	4. Most of the time
	5. All of the time
(10) Have you had any sudden, severe pain—'shooting', 'stabbing' or 'spasms'—from the affected hip?	1. No days
	2. Only 1 or 2 days
	3. Some days
	4. Most days
	5. Every day
(11) How much has pain from your hip interfered with your usual work (including housework)?	1. Not at all
	2. A little bit
	3. Moderately
	4. Greatly
	5. Totally
(12) Have you been troubled by pain from your hip in bed at night?	1. No nights
	2. Only 1 or 2 nights
	3. Some nights
	4. Most nights
	5. Every night

and EQ-VAS is 0.64 (Table 11.7) The figures for knees are: 2.23, 0.38, 0.39 (Table 11.8). An ES of 0.5 is a reasonable first approximation to a threshold for important change. This is supported by research in psychology that has shown that the limits of people's ability to discriminate is about this level [22].

Hip and knee replacement surgery is widely accepted by patients and surgeons as being highly beneficial, so it is surprising and of concern that the three measures do not agree. ES as measured by the Oxford scores is well above the 0.5 criterion for both hips and knees, but change measured by EQ-Index and EQ-VAS is around that figure.

The proportion of missing values is an indicator of how easy and relevant patients found it to complete the measure. The missing value rates for EQ-5D-3L are much higher than for the Oxford measures.

Table 11.7 Oxford Hip Score, EQ-5D Index and EQ-5D VAS before, after and change (0–100 scale, source NHS PROMs 2019–20)

	Hip replacement			
	Mean	SD	n	Missing (%)
Oxford score pre-op	36.4	17.1	21,351	1.0
Oxford score post-op	83.2	17.9	21,356	1.0
Oxford score change	46.8	21.1	21,147	2.0
EQ-index pre-op	58.5	57.6	20,344	6.0
EQ-index post-op	87.5	52.4	20,698	4.2
EQ-index change	28.9	21.6	19,557	10.3
EQ-VAS pre-op	63.3	22.1	19,743	9.2
EQ-VAS post-op	77.5	17.7	20,608	4.7
EQ-VAS change	14.1	23.6	18,938	13.9

Table 11.8 Oxford Knee Score, EQ-5D Index and EQ-5D VAS before, after and change (0–100 scale, source NHS PROMs 2019–20)

	Knee replacement			
	Mean	SD	n	Missing (%)
Oxford score pre-op	39.6	16.2	24,031	1.0
Oxford score post-op	75.7	19.4	23,883	1.6
Oxford score change	36.1	20.5	23,651	2.6
EQ-index pre-op	62.9	56.9	22,960	5.7
EQ-index post-op	84.5	52.8	23.381	3.8
EQ-index change	21.4	20.5	22,154	9.5
EQ-VAS pre-op	67.4	20.4	22,167	9.5
EQ-VAS post-op	75.3	17.8	23,351	3.9
EQ-VAS change	7.9	21.1	21,411	13.3

Correlations

Table 11.9 shows correlations between the Oxford hip and knee scores, EQ-Index and EQ-VAS before the operation (pre-op) and for change six months later. Note the relatively low correlations for both pre-operation ratings and change between EQ-VAS and both EQ-Index and Oxford scores (OHS and OKS). A correlation of $r=0.3$ only explains 9% of the variance.

Table 11.9 Pearson correlations between Oxford scores, EQ-5D Index and EQ-5D VAS for hip and knee replacements before surgery and for change before and after

	Hip replacement		Knee replacement	
	EQ-Index	EQ-VAS	EQ-Index	EQ-VAS
Pre-op				
Oxford score	0.73	0.39	0.70	0.38
EQ-Index		0.37		0.36
Post-op				
Oxford score	0.73	0.57	0.75	0.57
EQ-Index		0.63		0.61
Change				
Oxford score	0.64	0.35	0.60	0.32
EQ-index		0.34		0.30

Comparisons

For each measure described in this chapter, the number of items and response options, word count, Flesch-Kincaid readability grade (FKG) and range are shown in Table 11.10. This indicates differences in the design of each measure.

Word count and FKG include the items, preamble, and options of the versions found on referenced web sites, excluding the title or any copyright notices. Repeated options are only counted once. FKG was calculated using the *reading-formulas.com* web site. Reading age is approximately FKG + 5.

Table 11.10 Comparison of health status measures, showing, recall period, number of response options, word count, Flesch-Kincaid Grade (FKG) readability measure and possible range

Measure	Items	Options	Recall	Words	FKG	Range
SF-36 v2	36	2–6	4 weeks	650	4.3	PCS, MCS mean = 50, SD = 10
SF-12 v2	12	2–6	4 weeks	409	4.6	PCS, MCS mean = 50, SD = 10
EQ-5D-3L	5	3	Now	215	4.7	Index -0.59 to 1.0, VAS 0 to 100
EQ-5D-5L	5	5	Now	286	5.5	Index -0.59 to 1.0, VAS 0 to 100
howRu	4	4	1 day	31	1.6	0 to 100
OHS	12	5	4 weeks	420	3.3	12 to 60 (high is bad)
OKS	12	5	4 weeks	419	3.2	12 to 60 (high is bad)

The scoring schemes used vary.

- The SF measures use norm-based scoring based on the mean value of a population sample being 50 for both physical (PCS) and mental (MCS) components, with 10 points representing one standard deviation.
- EQ-5D uses a preference-based index score for the descriptive framework, based on ideal health valued as 1.0, dead 0 and a minimum score which may be negative. The visual analogue scale (EQ-VAS) has a range 0 to 100.
- The Oxford hip (OHS) and knee (OKS) scores report severity as high, with a range of 12 to 60 (worst state).

Conclusions

The primary purpose of health and care services is to improve the present and future health status of patients.

This chapter describes three generic measures designed to measure health status, SF-36 (and its derivative SF-12), EQ-5D and *howRu*. Two condition-specific measures (Oxford Hip Score and Oxford Knee Score) are also described.

References

1. Smith P (chair). NHS outcomes, performance and productivity: report of the Office of Health Economics commission. London: OHE; 2008.
2. Greenhalgh J. The applications of PROs in clinical practice: what they do, do they work, and why? Quality Life Res. 2009; 18:115–23.
3. Frost MH, Bonomi AE, Cappelleri JC, et al. Applying quality-of-life data formally and systematically into clinical practice. Mayo Clin Proc. 2007;82:1214–28.
4. Ware JE, Sherbourne CD. The MOS 36-item short-form health survey (SF-36). I. Conceptual framework and item selection. Med Care. 1992; 30:473–83.
5. Ware JE, Kosinski M, Keller SD. A 12-item short-form health survey: construction of scales and preliminary tests of reliability and validity. Med Care. 1996;34:220–33.
6. Brazier J, Ratcliffe J, Salomon JA, Tsuchiya A. Measuring and valuing health benefits for economic evaluation, 2nd ed. Oxford University Press; 2016.
7. Brooks RG. EuroQoL—the current state of play. Health Policy. 1996;37:53–72.
8. Szende A, Oppe M, Devlin N (eds.) EQ-5D value sets: inventory, comparative review and user guide. Euroqol Group Monographs, vol. 2, Dordrecht: Springer; 2007.
9. Dolan P. Modeling valuations for EuroQol health states. Med Care. 1997;35(11):1095–108.
10. Herdman M, Gudex C, Lloyd A, et al. Development and preliminary testing of the new five-level version of EQ-5D (EQ-5D-5L). Qual Life Res. 2011;20(10):1727–36.
11. Devlin N, Shah K, Feng Y, et al. Valuing health-related quality of life: an EQ-5D-5L value set for England. Health Econ. 2018;27(1):7–22.
12. Walloo A, Alva MH, Pudney S, et al. An international comparison of EQ-5D-5L and EQ-5D-3L for use in cost-effectiveness analysis. Value Health. 2021;24(4):568–74.
13. Benson T, Sizmur S, Whatling J, et al. Evaluation of a new short generic measure of health status: *howRu*. Inform Prim Care. 2010;18:89–101.
14. Rosser RM, Watts VC. The measurement of hospital output. Int J Epidemiol. 1972;1(4):361–8.

15. Stull DE, Leidy NK, Parasuraman P, Chassany O. Optimal recall periods for patient-reported outcomes: challenges and potential solutions. Curr Med Res Opin. 2009;25:929–42.
16. Streiner DL, Norman GR, Cairney J. Health measurement scales: a practical guide to their development and use, 5th ed. Oxford University Press; 2015.
17. https://files.digital.nhs.uk/1F/51FEDE/PROMs%20CSV%20Data%20Pack%20Provisional%201920.zip. Accessed 9 Sep 2021.
18. Benson T, Williams DH, Potts HWW. Performance of EQ-5D, howRu and Oxford Hip & Knee Scores in assessing the outcome of hip and knee replacements. BMC Health Serv Res. 2016;16:512.
19. Dawson J, Fitzpatrick R, Carr A, Murray D. Questionnaire on the perceptions of patients about total hip replacement. J Bone Joint Surg (Br). 1996;78(2):185–90.
20. Dawson J, Fitzpatrick R, Murray D, et al. Questionnaire on the perceptions of patients about total knee replacement. J Bone Joint Surg (Br). 1998;80(1):63–9.
21. Cohen J. Statistical power analysis for the behavioural sciences, 2nd ed. Hillsdale NJ: Lawrence Erlbaum; 1988.
22. Norman G, Sloan J, Wyrwich K. Interpretation of changes in health-related quality of life: the remarkable universality of half a standard deviation. Med Care. 2003;41(5):582–92.

Wellbeing 12

Background

The World Health Organization defines health as *a state of complete physical, mental and social wellbeing and not merely the absence of disease or infirmity* [1]. This definition has withstood the test of time well; many people equate health with wellbeing. The difficulties arise when we try to measure either health or wellbeing in a practical way.

In 2008, Nicholas Sarkozy, then President of the French Republic, set up a commission under the leadership of Joseph Stiglitz, Amartya Sen and Jean Paul Fitoussi to: Identify the limits of GDP as an indicator of economic performance and social progress, including the problems with its measurement; Consider what additional information might be required for the production of more relevant indicators of social progress; Assess the feasibility of alternative measurement tools; and Discuss how to present the statistical information in an appropriate way.

The unifying theme of the final report, published in 2009 was that the time was ripe for our measurement system to *shift emphasis from measuring economic production to measuring people's wellbeing* (original italics) [2]. A key recommendation was that national statistical offices should take the lead in measuring subjective wellbeing in population surveys.

Subjective Wellbeing

Subjective wellbeing (SWB) is synonymous with happiness and personal well-being. SWB refers to how people experience and evaluate their lives and specific domains and activities in their lives [3]. Measures of SWB aim to capture both pleasure and purpose in everyday life. Only the person involved can provide information about his or her SWB.

SWB is a multi-dimensional construct that is broader than just happiness or satisfaction. People need a sense of fulfilment and purpose as well. SWB has several facets:

- Evaluative wellbeing or life satisfaction.
- Eudemonic wellbeing—a sense of purpose and meaning in life.
- Affect or hedonistic wellbeing including both positive experiences, such as happiness, and negative experiences, such as anxiety.

People with high SWB are in general blessed with a positive temperament, look on the bright side of things, do not worry excessively about bad events, live in an economically developed society, have social confidants and adequate resources for making progress towards valued goals [4].

SWB differs in important ways from health status discussed in Chap. 11. The concept of evaluative wellbeing covers one's whole life, not just how you feel now and what you can do. Similarly, eudemonic wellbeing covers one's sense of purpose, which is essential if people are to flourish and feel content. People seek purpose in life as well as pleasure [5].

SWB focuses on what people feel, rather than function. People adapt less well to feeling miserable than to having a disability. After a time people think less about what they cannot do (disability) but find it hard not to ignore how you feel (distress). This focusing effect explains why getting old, buying a new car or moving to a sunny climate is often not as big a deal as you expect it to be in advance [6].

SWB has a U-shape for different ages, with a peak as a young adult, dip in middle age and then gradual improvement. This is unlike health status, which tends to fall as people get older and is the opposite of value of statistical life (VSL—see Chap. 8), which has an inverse U shape.

The Stiglitz-Sen-Fitoussi report created much interest internationally. In the UK, the Office of National Statistics (ONS) set up a Measuring National Wellbeing (MNW) programme in 2010, which among other objectives set out to measure SWB nationally [7].

ONS4

The ONS sought recommendations about questions that could be used to monitor progress, inform policy design and for policy appraisal [8]. They sought questions that could be added to existing surveys and could be answered quite quickly on paper, face-to-face or by telephone. They used the term *personal wellbeing* as being clearer and simpler to understand than subjective wellbeing.

Subjective Wellbeing

The final set, known as ONS4, is shown as Table 12.1 [9].

ONS4 has been a harmonised standard since 2015. These questions are used in more than 30 national surveys, enabling trends and comparisons to be seen.

When all four questions cannot be used, then *life satisfaction* and *worthwhileness* should be chosen. This is because they have the best correlation with the overall measure and relate to concepts that are measured internationally [10].

PWS

In 2015, I was asked to help evaluate an NHS Vanguard project with the brand name *Happy, Healthy at Home*. This led to the development of the Personal Wellbeing Score (PWS) [11].

The project team wanted a short easy to use measure of wellbeing to be used alongside other measures of patient experience (*howRwe*), health status (*howRu*), and health confidence (*HCS*). The *howRu* and *howRwe* measures have been described in Chaps. 10 and 11, and *HCS* is described in Chap. 13.

We evaluated the literature including ONS4 and the Short Warwick-Edinburgh Mental Well-Being Scale (SWEMWBS, see below) and after encouraging discussions with ONS, decided to adapt ONS4 to fit the format of the other measures. This involved several changes.

We felt that the wording used in ONS4 was unnecessarily verbose; we did not like that three questions were worded positively and one negatively, nor that it was recommended not to produce a single summary score. We also wanted a shorter set of response options.

A key change was the nature of the scale, from a numeric scale from 0 to 10, anchored at *not at all* (0) and *completely* (10) to four agree-disagree categories (*Strongly agree*, *Agree*, *Neutral* and *Disagree*). This was not as big a change as it sounds, because ONS report their own results in four groups, which correspond roughly to the four groups in PWS. The ONS life satisfaction, worthwhile and happiness scores are reported as: 9–10 *Very high*, 7–8 *High*, 5–6 *Medium* and 0–4 *Low*.

We changed the direction of the question on anxiety from negative (*Overall, how anxious did you feel yesterday?*) to positive (*I was NOT anxious yesterday*).

Table 12.1 ONS4 Personal Wellbeing Questions showing the suggested introduction and the four questions	Next, I would like to ask you four questions about your feelings on aspects of your life. There are no right or wrong answers. For each of these questions I'd like you to give an answer on a scale of 0–10, where 0 is "not at all" and 10 is "completely"
	Overall, how satisfied are you with your life nowadays?
	Overall, to what extent do you feel the things you do in your life are worthwhile?
	Overall, how happy did you feel yesterday?
	On a scale where 0 is "not at all anxious" and 10 is "completely anxious", overall, how anxious did you feel yesterday?

The word NOT is usually written in capital letters. There is no good English word meaning "not anxious" and having all items positively worded provides greater consistency, simpler scoring and easier reporting.

In testing, we found that exploratory factor analysis shows that all items in PWS relate to the same construct, inter-item correlations are in the range 0.51–0.77 and Cronbach's $\alpha = 0.90$ indicates that it is appropriate to aggregate individual item scores to generate a single summary score [12].

On the other hand, exploratory factor analysis of ONS4 data suggests that the negatively worded anxiety question is related to a different factor than the three positively worded questions. This is one reason why ONS do not recommend aggregating the item scores to produce a single summary score. This is also found in other measures that have positively and negatively worded items [13].

As with other R-Outcomes measures, colour-coded emoji are used. *Strongly agree* is a green grin, *Agree* is a yellow smile, *Neutral* is a straight-mouth orange and *Disagree* is red sad.

These changes reduced the word count and the reading age.

The scoring scheme used for PWS is similar to that used for the *howRu* health status measure, described in Chap. 11. At the individual level, the four items are scored from 0 (Disagree) to 3 (Strongly agree). A summary score is calculated with a range from 0 to 12 by aggregating the item scores. At the population level, mean scores are calculated by converting all scales to a common 0 to 100 scale.

The summary score is not calculated for responses with any missing item values. This is usually under 2% of responses.

The final version of PWS is shown in Fig. 12.1.

EQ Health and Wellbeing

The EQ Health and Wellbeing (EQ-HWB) is a new generic measure, which includes aspects of wellbeing such as autonomy and relationships that are important to patients and care users. The full EQ-HWB has 25 items and a short version (EQ-HWB-S) has 9 items covering mobility, daily activities, coping, concentration and thinking clearly, anxiety, sad/depression, loneliness, fatigue and pain. It has been developed internationally for evaluating interventions in health, public health and social care including the impact on patients, social care users and carers [14].

Mental Health

The mental health services have always shown most interest in measuring wellbeing, due in part to the relative lack of suitable laboratory and imaging tests for mental health and reliance on what the patient says.

Here we describe on two tools aimed at the mild end of the mental health spectrum, WEMWBS and ReQoL. Both use simple language and are relatively quick and easy to use.

Mental Health

Personal Wellbeing

How are you feeling in general?

	Strongly agree	Agree	Neutral	Disagree
I am satisfied with my life	😀	🙂	😐	☹️
What I do in my life is worthwhile	😀	🙂	😐	☹️
I was happy yesterday	😀	🙂	😐	☹️
I was NOT anxious yesterday	😀	🙂	😐	☹️

Fig. 12.1 Personal Wellbeing Score (PWS)

WEMWBS

WEMWBS (Warwick-Edinburgh Mental Well-Being Scale) focuses on mental wellbeing. The concept of mental wellbeing is broader than the absence of diagnosed mental illness or psychiatric disorders.

WEMWBS has 14 items with 5 response options each. Item scores are summed to provide a single summary score with a range from 14 to 70 [14]. There is also a short version with seven items, SWEMWBS (Short Warwick-Edinburgh Mental Well-Being Scale), with a range from 7 to 35 [15]. See Table 12.2.

The options are: *None of the time, Rarely, Some of the time, Often and All of the time, scored from 1 to 5 respectively*. A high score is good. All items are all worded positively, use simple language and cover both feelings and functional aspects of mental wellbeing.

ReQoL

Recovering Quality of Life (ReQoL) is a generic self-reported outcome measure for use with people experiencing mental health difficulties [16]. It is designed to help service users in their recovery journey and to feel more in control of what happens with their treatment by showing their progress.

ReQoL has two versions. The first 10 items of the longer version (ReQoL-20) are the same as the shorter version (ReQoL-10). Both versions include positively and negatively worded items. The five response options are: *None of the time, only occasionally, sometimes, often and most of the time*. These are scored on a 0–4 scale where a high score is good (Table 12.3).

For ReQoL-10, the range of scores is 0 to 40. The minimally important difference (MID) is 5 points, which means that a patient improvement or deterioration of

Table 12.2 Warwick-Edinburgh Mental Well-Being Scale (WEMWBS). © NHS Health Scotland, University of Warwick and University of Edinburgh, 2008, all rights reserved

WEMWBS	SWEMWBS (*)
Below are some statements about feelings and thoughts. Please tick the box that best describes your experience of each over the last 2 weeks	*
I've been feeling useful	*
I've been feeling relaxed	*
I've been feeling interested in other people	
I've had energy to spare	
I've been dealing with problems well	*
I've been thinking clearly	*
I've been feeling good about myself	
I've been feeling close to other people	*
I've been feeling confident	
I've been able to make up my own mind about things	*
I've been feeling loved	
I've been interested in new things	
I've been feeling cheerful	

more than 5 points is reliable, but less than 5 points is not. Scores between 25 and 40 are normal (within the range of the general population). Scores below 25 are clinically important. For ReQoL-20 these scores are doubled.

Historically, most measures used in mental health have focused on clinical diagnosis. For example, they may be designed to collect the diagnosis criteria listed in the American Psychiatric Association's diagnostic and statistical manual of mental disorders (DSM-5) [17]. This approach is designed less to help service users get better than to help clinicians classify them correctly. This may be a preparatory step to arranging help. Furthermore, many widely used measures focus on only one symptom or diagnosis, such as depression (PHQ-9) [18] or anxiety (GAD-7) [19].

Comparisons

Table 12.4 compares the word count, Flesch-Kincaid readability grade (FKG), the number of positively and negatively worded items and the range of scores possible for a group of people for each measure described in this chapter. This shows differences in the design of each measure.

Word count and FKG include the items, preamble, and options, but not the title or any copyright notices. FKG was calculated using the *readingformulas.com* web site. Reading age is approximately FKG + 5. Range is the possible score range of values from floor to ceiling. All wellbeing measures are positive (high is good).

Table 12.3 ReQoL™ Version 1.1 © Copyright, The University of Sheffield 2016, 2018. All Rights Reserved. The authors have asserted their moral rights. Oxford University Innovation Limited is exclusively licensed to grant permissions to use the ReQoL™

ReQoL-20	ReQoL-10 (*)	Positive (pos) or negative (neg)
For each of the following statements, please tick one box that best describes your thoughts, feelings and activities over the **last week**		
1. I found it difficult to get started with everyday tasks	*	neg
2. I felt able to trust others	*	pos
3. I felt unable to cope	*	neg
4. I could do the things I wanted to do	*	pos
5. I felt happy	*	pos
6. I thought my life was not worth living	*	neg
7. I enjoyed what I did	*	pos
8. I felt hopeful about my future	*	pos
9. I felt lonely	*	neg
10. I felt confident in myself	*	pos
11. I did things I found rewarding		pos
12. I avoided things I needed to do		neg
13. I felt irritated		neg
14. I felt like a failure		neg
15. I felt in control of my life		pos
16. I felt terrified		neg
17. I felt anxious		neg
18. I had problems with my sleep		neg
19. I felt calm		pos
20. I found it hard to concentrate		neg
Please describe your physical health (problems with pain, mobility, difficulties caring for yourself or feeling physically unwell) **over the last week**	*	neg

Table 12.4 Comparison of wellbeing measures showing: recall period, number of response options, word count, Flesch-Kincaid Grade (FKG), number of positively and negatively worded items, and score range for groups of people

Measure	Items	Options	Recall period	Word count	FKG	Positive items	Negative items	Range
ONS4	4	11	1 day	107	6.1	3	1	0 to 10
PWS	4	4	1 day	34	4.3	4	–	0 to 100
WEMWBS	14	5	2 weeks	117	3.4	14	–	14 to 70
SWEMWBS	7	5	2 weeks	81	2.9	7	–	7 to 35
ReQoL-20	20	5	1 week	164	3.8	9	11	0 to 80
ReQoL-10	10	5	1 week	115	4.6	6	4	0 to 40

References

1. Constitution of the World Health Organization. Geneva: WHO; 1948.
2. Stiglitz J, Sen A, Fitoussi J-P. Report by the commission on the measurement of economic performance and social progress; 2009 www.stiglitz-sen-fitoussi.fr.
3. Steptoe A, Deaton A, Stone A. Subjective wellbeing, health, and ageing. Lancet. 2015;385 (9968):640–8.
4. Diener E, Suh E, Lucas R, Smith H. Subjective well-being: three decades of research. Psychol Bull. 1999;125(2):276–302.
5. Dolan P. Happiness by design: finding pleasure and purpose in everyday life. London: Allen Lane; 2014.
6. Schkade D, Kahneman D. Does living in California make people happy: a focussing illusion in judgments of life satisfaction. Psychol Sci. 1998;9(5):340–6.
7. Allin P, Hand D. New statistics for old?—measuring the wellbeing of the UK. J R Statist Soc A. 2017;180:3–43.
8. Dolan P, Layard R, Metcalfe R. Measuring subjective wellbeing for public policy: recommendations on measures. Special paper 23. Centre for Economic Performance, London School of Economics and Political Science; 2011.
9. Nickson S. Personal wellbeing harmonised standard. London: Government Statistical Service; 2020. https://gss.civilservice.gov.uk/policy-store/personal-well-being/. Accessed 14 Sept 2021.
10. VanderWeele T, Trudel-Fitzgerald C, Allin P, et al. Current recommendations on the selection of measures for well-being. Preven Med. 2020; 133:106004.
11. Benson T, Sladen J, Liles A, Potts, HW. Personal Wellbeing Score (PWS)—a short version of ONS4: development and validation in social prescribing. BMJ Open Qual. 2019; 8(2): e000394.
12. Streiner DL, Norman GR, Cairney J. Health measurement scales: a practical guide to their development and use. 5th edition. Oxford University Press; 2015.
13. Mukuria C, Rowen D, Peasgood T, Brazier J. An empirical comparison of well-being measures used in the UK. Policy Res Unit Econ Evalu Health Soc Care Interven (EEPRU) (27); 2016.
14. Brazier J, Peasgood T, Mukaria C, et al. The EQ Health and Wellbeing: Overview of the Development of a Measure ofHealth and Wellbeing and Key Results. Value in Health 2022 (in press) https://doi.org/10.1016/j.jval.2022.01.009
15. Stewart-Brown S, Tennant A, Tennant R, et al. Internal construct validity of the Warwick-Edinburgh mental well-being scale (WEMWBS): a Rasch analysis using data from the Scottish health education population survey. Health Qual Life Outcomes. 2009;7:1–8.
16. Keetharuth AD, Brazier J, Connell J, et al. Recovering Quality of Life (ReQoL): a new generic self-reported outcome measure for use with people experiencing mental health difficulties. Br J Psychiat. 2018;212:42–9.
17. American Psychiatric Association. Diagnostic and statistical manual of mental disorders, 5th ed. Arlington: American Psychiatric Association; 2013.
18. Kroenke K, Spitzer R, Williams J. The PHQ-9. J Gen Intern Med. 2001;16:606–13.
19. Spitzer R, Kroenke K, Williams JB, Löwe B. A brief measure for assessing generalized anxiety disorder: the GAD-7. Arch Intern Med. 2006;166:1092–7.

Patient-Centred Care

Patient-Centered Care

Patient-centered care, also known as personalised care, means making the patients' needs and wishes paramount. This differs from the traditional medical model which is focused on what is the matter with the patient, as opposed to what matters to the patient.

The patient-centered care approach has led to three new roles: health coaches who help people improve their ability to look after themselves, link workers who link patients with voluntary and other non-medical support services in the community, and care coordinators who help orchestrate services for people living with multiple long-term conditions.

People living with chronic conditions make many day-to-day decisions about their illnesses. They self-manage. Recognition of this fact leads to a new need for collaborative care or shared decision-making, and self-management education [1]. Many people have problems that are a complex mix of medical, social and emotional issues, which are not amenable to drug prescriptions or a one-size-fits-all approach.

Self-management education supports patients to live the best possible quality of life with their chronic conditions. Whereas traditional patient education provides information and technical skills, self-management education teaches problem-solving, so they can look after themselves when possible.

Self-efficacy

A central idea in self-management is *self-efficacy*—the confidence to carry out the behaviour needed to reach a desired goal. Self-efficacy is enhanced when patients can solve problems that they themselves have identified. The term self-efficacy was promoted by psychologist Albert Bandura to describe a person's capacity to do what is needed to achieve specific tasks [2]. It is a general concept affecting all areas of human endeavor. Self-efficacy impacts the power a person has to face challenges competently and also the choices they make.

A strong sense of self-efficacy promotes accomplishment and personal well-being. People with high self-efficacy see challenges as things to overcome rather than threats to avoid. They recover from difficulties faster and are more likely to attribute failure to a lack of effort than anything inherent in the problem. They approach threatening situations believing that they can control them.

People with low self-efficacy shy away from hard tasks. They worry about their lack of skills rather than employ the ones they have. They lose faith in their own abilities after a setback. Low self-efficacy is linked to anxiety and depression.

Most health care policy aims to improve the cost-effectiveness of health care. A popular approach is to try to reduce the need for people to be admitted to hospitals, because that is where most of the money is spent. Ideally more people should self-manage their own health themselves.

Supported Self-management

Supported self-management includes all of the ways that health and care services encourage, support, and empower people to self-manage their ongoing physical and mental health conditions. People living with ongoing health conditions should be empowered to live well with their conditions [3]. In particular, patients need to develop confidence (self-efficacy) to look after themselves most of the time, but to know when to seek help if they need it.

The terms self-efficacy, self-management, patient activation, patient engagement and health confidence are often used interchangeably, although specialists discern distinctions. Here we use these terms as synonyms. We use the term self-efficacy to describe the overall construct.

Patients want to be actively engaged in their own care. One of the objectives of supported self-management is to help people to become as confident and self-efficacious as possible when confronted with ongoing health conditions and the challenges they bring. To do this we need to measure self-efficacy, so we know how they are doing and can help most effectively. People on different parts of the self-efficacy spectrum respond best to different types of help.

Measures of self-efficacy are sensitive to each person's health problems and how these change over time. For example, a person with no long-term health problems will usually score better than a person living with multiple problems. Case-mix, health status and social status must all be considered, so we compare like with like.

It is easier to boost self-efficacy for people who start from a low point than for those starting higher up. When someone with high self-efficacy has a setback, it may be a good result if they maintain their level. Measurement needs to become an integral part of a process to support and tailor person-centred care, not just to measure its success.

Self-efficacy is primarily a mind-set, but health literacy (understanding health literature) is a skill set, which is different. There is only a weak relationship between mind-sets and skill sets, although one way to improve the former is to ensure that people know how to do what they need to do [4].

Measures

Evidence suggests that programs designed to improve self-efficacy frequently improve outcomes and lower costs [1, 5]. Measures of self-efficacy and self-management capability may be used at the individual, service or population level. They can be used to tailor care to individual needs, measure outcomes, help us understand whether interventions reach and help their target participants, or whether we are only reaching those with already high self-efficacy.

This section describes three measures which have been designed to measure self-efficacy for use in self-management: the Patient Activation Measure (PAM), My Health Confidence (MHC) and the Health Confidence Score (HCS).

Patient Activation Measure (PAM)

The Patient Activation Measure (PAM) was one of the first measures of its type to be developed for use in healthcare. Patient activation is defined as understanding one's role in the care process and having the knowledge skills and confidence to manage one's health and healthcare.

The original version had 22 items (PAM-22) [6]. This was followed by a short-form version (PAM-13) with 13 items [7]. The version of PAM-13 mainly used in the UK shown in Table 13.1.

Patient activation emphasises patients' ability and willingness to act independently to manage their health and care. It differs from compliance, which is about getting patients to follow medical advice.

In general people with higher activation are more likely to self-manage their conditions when not being treated, feel confident in managing their own health and play a more active role in staying healthy. They seek help when they need it and actively think about their health and make more informed choices. All this leads to better outcomes in terms of higher quality of life, greater satisfaction with the care they get and use of less healthcare resources [5].

PAM is particularly relevant for people living with long-term conditions.

There are three types of PAM score. The raw score is the sum of the 13 item scores, each scored 1–4, giving a range from 13 to 52. These scores are then transformed using a secret algorithm to an individual patient activation score on a 0–100 scale (where high is good). They are also grouped into four activation levels:

Level 1: Disengaged and overwhelmed
Level 2: Becoming aware but still struggling
Level 3: Taking action
Level 4: Maintaining behaviours and pushing further.

Table 13.1 Patient activation measure (PAM-13) UK Version © 2019 Insignia Health. All rights reserved. Response options: Disagree strongly; Disagree; Agree; Agree strongly; N/A

Your answers to the following questions will help us provide the support that is right for you. Please indicate how much you agree or disagree with each statement as it applies to you personally. Many people find that they do not agree with all the statements, which is normal. There are no right or wrong answers, just answer with what is true for you
1. I am the person who is responsible for taking care of my health
2. Taking an active role in my own health care is the most important thing that affects my health
3. I am confident I can help prevent or reduce problems associated with my health
4. I know what each of my prescribed medications do
5. I am confident that I can tell whether I need to go to the doctor or whether I can take care of a health problem myself
6. I am confident that I can tell a doctor or nurse concerns I have even when he or she does not ask
7. I am confident that I can carry out medical treatments I may need to do at home
8. I understand my health problems and what causes them
9. I know what treatments are available for my health problems
10. I have been able to maintain lifestyle changes, like healthy eating or exercising
11. I know how to prevent problems with my health
12. I am confident I can work out solutions when new problems arise with my health
13. I am confident that I can maintain lifestyle changes, like healthy eating and exercising, even during times of stress

My Health Confidence

My Health Confidence (MHC) is a direct measure of self-care confidence [8]. MHC has two questions answered on a scale from 0 to 10 (11 points). The end points are indicated by green grin and sad red emojis (Table 13.2). The scores for each item are reported separately.

Table 13.2 My health confidence items

Item
1. *MHC Confidence.* How confident are you that you can control and manage most of your health problems?
2. *MHC Information.* How understandable and useful is the information that your doctors and nurses have given you about your health problems or concerns?

Health Confidence

How do you feel about caring for your health?

	Strongly agree	Agree	Neutral	Disagree
I know enough about my health	🙂	🙂	😐	☹️
I can look after my health	🙂	🙂	😐	☹️
I can get the right help when I need it	🙂	🙂	😐	☹️
I am involved in decisions about me	🙂	🙂	😐	☹️

Fig. 13.1 Health Confidence Score (HCS)

Health Confidence Score (HCS)

When we decided to develop a measure of personal well-being (see Chap. 11), we also identified the need for a short broad generic measure of patients' own perception of their health confidence, for use in quality improvement, impact evaluation and tailoring individual care. We called this the Health Confidence Score (HCS) [9].

Design criteria were to be clear, short with a low reading age. The measure needed to be used alongside other PROMs and PREMs, such as *howRu* (Chap. 11), *PWS* (Chap. 12) and *howRwe* (Chap. 10), so we used the same format and scoring scheme (Fig. 13.1).

HCS is broader and shorter than other measures covering aspects of health knowledge, access to care and shared decision-making as well as self-management.

It has four dimensions:

Knowledge—This is about how much the patient understands about their conditions and treatment, including health literacy. *I know enough about my health.*

Self-management—This is the patient's perceived ability to manage his or her own conditions, treatment and lifestyle. *I can look after my health.*

Access—This covers the patient's social proficiency to navigate the health system to obtain the services needed. *I can get the right help if I need it.*

Shared decision-making—This covers the patient's participation in clinical decisions and how well staff understand his or her wishes. A more detailed Shared Decisions measure is described below. *I am involved in decisions about me.*

Discussion

The choice of these dimensions was influenced by Michie's COM-B model, [10] which is described under Behaviour Change in Chaps. 4 and 16. In summary, all behaviour change depends on people's capability, opportunity, and motivation to change what they do.

I know enough about my health relates to capability and how people understand how their behaviour impacts their health.

I can look after my health is about self-efficacy and has aspects of both capability and motivation; they may not be able to change things or may not wish to change.

I can get the right help if I need it and *I am involved in decisions that affect me* relate to opportunity and how local health and care services help and support them.

The focus is on how people feel (their mind-set), not on what they do. Most people who smoke know it is bad for them but do it anyway. Health confidence is about each patient's perception of themselves, not a clinical encounter, nor about how well clinicians engage with them, which is often the focus of initiatives to improve shared decision-making.

Case Study

In this case study 381 people completed a short survey, which included HCS, MHC, the *howRu* health status measure (described in Chap. 11) and demographic details including gender, age in deciles, ethnicity, children (y/n), number of medications taken, education level and English region. The sample is from a convenience sample of the general population in southern England; most people were in good health. Full details of this study have been published [9].

The frequency distribution for HCS items is shown in Table 13.3. Cronbach's $\alpha = 0.82$, which indicates that it is appropriate to aggregate the item scores into a single aggregate score. Internal inter-item correlations were all in the range 0.41 to 0.59 indicating that each item measures different but related things. This confirms that it is useful to look at each item independently and also to aggregate them as a summary score.

The mean aggregate HCS score (sum of the four individual item scores) was 76.7 (SD = 20.4) when transposed to 0–100 scale. 23% of ratings were at the ceiling (Strongly agree on all four items) and only one (0.3%) at the floor.

The MHC confidence scores were 8.4 (SD = 1.3). For comparability with HCS, multiply by 10. Smaller standard deviation indicates that MHC confidence has a narrower (spikier) distribution than HCS.

Table 13.3 Frequency distribution of HCS items (n = 381)

HCS Item	Strongly agree (%)	Agree (%)	Neutral (%)	Disagree (%)
I know enough about my health	43	45	10	2
I can look after my health	40	39	17	3
I can get the right help if I need it	50	40	8	1
I am involved in decisions about me	53	32	12	4

Spearman correlations between HCS and MHC confidence scores were highly correlated r = 0.76. HCS is moderately correlated with *howRu* health status (r = 0.49), weakly negatively correlated with age group (r = –0.22) and number of medications taken (r = –0.29). Health confidence tends to fall as people acquire more health problems. HCS is not significantly correlated with the MHC Information scores (r = 0.08) nor significantly associated with ethnicity, having children, education level or English region.

Exploratory factor analysis confirms that HCS measures the same construct as MHC Confidence, but *howRu* and the MHC Information item measure different things.

In this study, all of the findings were as expected, providing evidence of construct validity for the health confidence score (HCS).

Comparison of Measures

Table 13.4 compares the number of items, number of response options, word count, Flesch-Kincaid readability grade (FKG), and the range of scores possible for a group of people for each measure described in this chapter. This shows differences in the design of each measure. A high score is good for all measures.

Word count and FKG include the standard items, preamble, and options, but not the title or any copyright notices. FKG was calculated using the readingformulas.com web site. Reading age is approximately FKG + 5. Range is the possible score range of values from floor to ceiling.

Shared Decision-Making

Shared decision-making (SDM) is a collaborative process that involves a person and their healthcare professional working together to reach a joint decision about care. It could be care or treatment the person needs straightaway or in the future, for example, through advance care planning.

The benefits of SDM are to allow people to discuss and share information to ensure that they have a good understanding of the benefits, harms and possible outcomes of different options.

Table 13.4 Comparison of measures showing: number of items, number of response options, recall period, word count, Flesch-Kincaid Grade (FKG) readability measure and possible range

Measure	Items	Options	Recall	Words	FKG	Range
PAM-13	13	4 + N/A	Now	280	4.4	0 to 100 + 4 levels
MHC	2	11	Now	42	5.4	0 to 10
HCS	4	4	Now	43	2.2	0 to 100

It empowers people to make decisions about what treatment and care is right for them at that time. This includes choosing to continue with their current treatment or choosing no treatment at all.

It allows people the opportunity to choose to what degree they want to engage in decision making. Some people prefer not to take an active role in making decisions with their healthcare professionals [11].

The General Medical Council in the UK have set out seven principles of decision-making and consent [12]:

1. All patients have the right to be involved in decisions about their treatment and care and be supported to make informed decisions if they are able.
2. Decision making is an ongoing process focused on meaningful dialogue: the exchange of relevant information specific to the individual patient.
3. All patients have the right to be listened to, and to be given the information they need to make a decision and the time and support they need to understand it.
4. Doctors must try to find out what matters to patients so they can share relevant information about the benefts and harms of proposed options and reasonable alternatives, including the option to take no action.
5. Doctors must start from the presumption that all adult patients have capacity to make decisions about their treatment and care. A patient can only be judged to lack capacity to make a specifc decision at a specifc time, and only after assessment in line with legal requirements.
6. The choice of treatment or care for patients who lack capacity must be of overall benefit to them, and decisions should be made in consultation with those who are close to them or advocating for them.
7. Patients whose right to consent is affected by law should be supported to be involved in the decision-making process, and to exercise choice if possible.

The SDM process may include: (1) Encouraging people to talk about what is important to them; communicating with people in a way they can understand, using clear language, avoiding jargon and explaining technical terms. (2) Sharing and discussing the information and evidence that people need to make informed decisions. (3) Making sure they understand the choices available to them, including the choice of doing nothing or not changing the current plan. (4) Communicating with and involving family members, friends, carers, advocates or other people who the person chooses to include. (5) Use of patient decision aids.

Clinical decisions can be complex and involve trade-offs between efficacy, safety, convenience and cost, as well as arcane terms, such as the names of drugs and procedures. For example, the difference between arthroplasty (joint replacement) and arthroscopy (joint investigation) is obvious to a surgeon, but not to the average patient. Making SDM work can be difficult.

There is still uncertainty about how best to measure SDM effectiveness [13]. Here, we discuss two measures. The CollaborRATE tool focuses on the SDM process; the Shared Decisions measure focuses more on SDM outcome.

CollaboRATE

The CollaborRATE tool is a short patient-completed measure of the SDM process [14]. Patients rate the extent to which their healthcare provider helped them to understand their health issue, listened to them and included them in the decision-making. It has three items, each rated on a 10-point scale from: 1 (no effort was made) to 10 (every effort was made).

1. How much effort was made to help you understand your health issues?
2. How much effort was made to listen to the things that matter most to you about your health issues?
3. How much effort was made to include what matters to you in choosing what to do next?

Here the focus is on how much effort patients think was made. This raises the old debate about process and outcomes. It is not inevitable that better process leads to better outcome.

Shared Decisions

The Shared Decisions measure focuses directly on patient perceptions of SDM results. These are often lacking [15]. It asks patients how much they understand the benefits and risks of the way forward (the plan), whether they understand that they have choices, and if they feel fully engaged in the decisions (see Fig. 13.2).

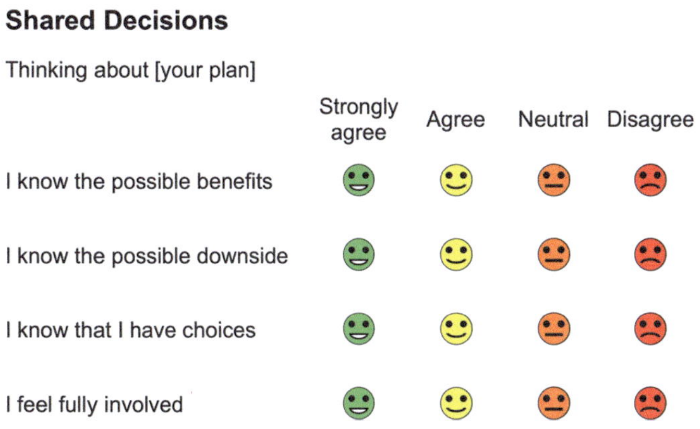

Shared Decisions

Thinking about [your plan]

	Strongly agree	Agree	Neutral	Disagree
I know the possible benefits	😀	🙂	😐	☹️
I know the possible downside	😀	🙂	😐	☹️
I know that I have choices	😀	🙂	😐	☹️
I feel fully involved	😀	🙂	😐	☹️

Fig. 13.2 Shared decisions measure

References

1. Bodenheimer T, Lorig K, Holman H, Grumbach K. Patient self-management of chronic disease in primary care. JAMA. 2002;288(19):2469–75.
2. Bandura A. Self-efficacy mechanism in human agency. Am Psychol. 1982;37(2):122–47.
3. NHS. The NHS long term plan; 2019. https://www.longtermplan.nhs.uk.
4. Smith SG, Curtis LM, Wardle J, et al. Skill set or mind set? Associations between health literacy, patient activation and health. PLOS One. 2013;8:e74373.
5. Hibbard JH, Greene J. What the evidence shows about patient activation: better health outcomes and care experiences; fewer data on costs. Health Aff. 2013;32(4):207–14.
6. Hibbard JH, Stockard J, Mahoney ER, Tusler M. Development of the patient activation measure (PAM): conceptualizing and measuring activation in patients and consumers. Health Serv Res. 2004;39(4 part 1):1005–26.
7. Hibbard JH, Mahoney ER, Stockard J, Tusler M. Development and testing of a short form of the patient activation measure. Health Serv Res. 2005;40(6 part 1):1918–30.
8. Wasson J, Coleman EA. Health confidence: a simple essential measure for patient engagement and better practice. Fam Pract Manag. 2014;21(5):8–12.
9. Benson T, Potts HWW, Bark P, Bowman C. Development and initial testing of a health confidence score (HCS). BMJ Open Qual. 2019;8:e000411.
10. Michie S, van Stralen MM, West R. The behaviour change wheel: A new method for characterising and designing behaviour change interventions. Implem Sci. 2011;6:42.
11. Coulter A, Collins A. Making shared decision-making a reality: no decision about me, without me. The Kings Fund; 2011.
12. Decision making and consent. General Medical Council 2020; GMC/DMC/0920
13. Shared decision-making. NICE Guideline NG197; 2021.
14. Barr PJ, Thompson R, Walsh T, et al. The psychometric properties of CollaboRATE: a fast and frugal patient-reported measure of the shared decision-making process. J Med Internet Res. 2014;16(1):e2.
15. Bomhof-Roordink H, Gärtner FR, Stiggelbout AM, et al. Key components of shared decision making models: a systematicreview. BMJ Open 2019; 9: e031763.

Individualised Measures

14

Background

As discussed in Chap. 1, patient-reported outcome and experience measures (PROMs and PREMs) fall into three broad categories:

- Condition-specific measures, which are applicable to patients with specific conditions only. Thousands of condition-specific measures have been developed mainly for use in clinical trials.
- Generic measures, which apply to all patient types. Standardised generic measures are widely used in evaluation, for quality improvement and for allocating resources between different groups.
- Individualised or person-specific measures (sometimes called iPROMs), which let people identify issues which are most important to them. Only a few individualised measures have been developed, although there is a new awareness of their value in tailoring personalised care in fields such as social prescribing.

To date, most uses of PROMs have been in research and to a lesser extent for monitoring the health of specific populations. Their use in routine clinical practice is relatively rare but the following key factors have been identified [1]:

1. Purpose of using the measure should be clear.
2. Measures used should be simple, valid, responsive, easy to interpret and relevant.
3. Setting chosen should be questionnaire friendly.
4. Feedback should be frequent and prompt.
5. Adequate support and training should be provided for patients and staff.

Most PROMs and PREMs are based on three assumptions: the same domains of life are important to all people; in each field people have the similar needs and goals; and success is related to the extent that these needs are satisfied, and goals met.

However, people differ greatly in how important they consider different things to be, individually and over time. For example, some people with disabilities adapt well to living with them, although others do not [2]. Individualised measures address this need.

Individualised Measures

The focus in personalised care is on the respondent and what matters to each individually, rather than what others think should matter most to them. Individualised measures can be used by patients and by staff. Patients expect that their individual needs and desires be recognised and fulfilled if possible. Individualised measures allow people to say in their own words what they need help with and to indicate how important each issue is.

Individualised measures help patients and healthcare professionals align priorities. Every person has their own priorities although some may be easier to help with than others. This applies across clinical, social and emotional issues.

Some conditions and issues will get better without help, some will stay the same and some will get worse. For this reason, individualised measures are usually used alongside generic or condition-specific measures of health status, wellbeing, health confidence and so on. When used in this way, individualised measures can be used to tailor patient-centred plans, goal setting and prioritisation, especially for people living with multiple problems.

Several individualised measures were developed during the 1990s, such as SEIQOL (Schedule for Evaluation of Individual Quality Of Life), [3] PGI (Patient Generated Index) [4] and MYMOP (Measure Yourself Medical Outcome Profile) [5]. However, the first generation of individualised measures proved to be hard to use and analyse [2].

MYCaW

Measure Yourself Concerns and Wellbeing (MYCaW) was developed from MYMOP to help evaluate cancer support services, where the need was for an outcome questionnaire that allowed for more holistic concerns, not just symptoms. It also needed to be valid, responsive to change, and easy to use and interpret. MYCaW is also used in social prescribing and personalised care services.

MYCaW is simpler than MYMOP, with two concerns plus well-being [6, 7]. It is also used by carers [8]. Participants nominate one or two concerns and score these concerns together with their general feeling of wellbeing using a seven-point (0–6) scale, where a high score is bad.

Participants usually complete a first form during their first consultation and a follow-up form after they have received tailored support. Additional data collected includes the date, demographic data, the type of consultation (face-to-face; video, phone call) and who completed the form (person, carer, professional).

The follow-up form also has additional open questions about other things affecting their health and the most important aspects of the treatment. Participants usually complete a first form before treatment and a follow-up form after treatment. For more information see https://www.meaningfulmeasures.co.uk.

Person-Specific Outcome

The Person-Specific Outcome (PSO) was developed as a short quick-to-use measure at the request of customers working in social prescribing projects [9]. The questions are typically asked at first meeting with the patient and on follow-up. The layout, showing both first meeting and follow-up questions, is shown in Fig. 14.1.

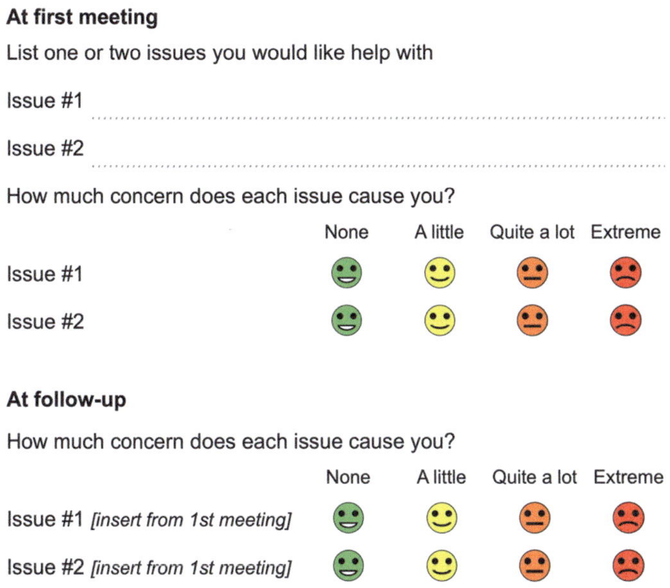
At first meeting

List one or two issues you would like help with

Issue #1 ....

Issue #2 ....

How much concern does each issue cause you?

	None	A little	Quite a lot	Extreme
Issue #1				
Issue #2				

At follow-up

How much concern does each issue cause you?

	None	A little	Quite a lot	Extreme
Issue #1 *[insert from 1st meeting]*				
Issue #2 *[insert from 1st meeting]*				

Fig. 14.1 Person specific outcome measure showing first meeting and follow-up questions

The PSO works in a similar way to other measures in the R-Outcomes family of short generic patient-reported outcome measures (PROMs) and patient-reported experience measures (PREMs). These common characteristics include [10]:

1. Brevity and low reading age
2. Quick and easy to use
3. Four response options
4. Optional use of emojis (smiley faces) and colour (green, yellow, orange red) to help understanding
5. Easy to interpret results
6. A high score is always good, low is bad. This means that improvement between first meeting and follow-up is shown as a positive number
7. Mean scores for a population are reported on 0 to 100 scale
8. Designed to be used together with other measures with the same characteristics.

On follow-up, the original issue(s) are pre-populated with the issue texts recorded at first meeting. Patient are asked to record their current level of concern. The questions can be asked face-to-face or by telephone. We do not recommend asking these questions at first meeting without any staff involvement, because patients often seek advice about what type of issues to record.

For individuals, the PSO uses the same response options as the *howRu* health status measure (see Chap. 11) [11]. *Extreme* scores 0, *Quite a lot* scores 1, *A little* scores 2 and *None* scores 3. In reports on individuals, the original patient-specific text and the response label (e.g., *Quite a lot*) and or score is used for each issue.

When reporting the results for a cohort, the mean scores for Issue #1 and Issue #2 are presented on a 0–100 scale (by multiplying by 100 and dividing by 3). Improvement is a positive number. Mean scores are usually shown without decimal points. A summary score is not calculated.

For example:

First meeting (Issue #1) mean score = 30
Follow-up (Issue #1) mean score = 70
Mean change (Issue #1) = 40

The PSO is short and easy to use, with four response options, which are labelled with words and coloured emojis, not numbers. Mean scores for a population are shown on a 0–100 scale with a high score always being high. This means that reported improvement is signified by a positive number. A summary score is not generated.

Individualised outcome measures are useful when people are living with multiple long-term conditions, and it is important to help them adapt. They help health and care staff identify and tailor support to what matters most to their patients. They can identify specific improvements to peoples' quality of life, even if they cannot modify the natural history of disease or other underlying problems.

In some areas it is appropriate to suggest that patients list issues that staff may be expected to help them with, rather than long-term medical issues or economic issues that are outside of their scope.

However, because people can prioritise very different things, these tools should be used together with generic PROMs and PREMs. Unpublished findings suggest that changes in PSO scores correlate strongly with changes in well-being as measured by the Personal Well-being Score (PWS), [12] but not with changes in health status [11] nor health confidence [13].

The main technical issue in using individualised measures, is to digitally pre-populate the follow-up survey with the issues recorded on the initial survey for the same patient. This needs some form of patient identifier and specialised software.

Changes identified by individualised outcome measures are often large, but must be interpreted with caution. A large improvement means that the specific issue has been resolved. Such improvements are extremely worthwhile, but do not mean that patients have recovered from their underlying disease or diseases.

Comparisons

Table 14.1 compares the number of items, number of response options, word count, Flesch-Kincaid readability grade (FKG), and the range of scores possible for a group of people for each measure using the text shown in this chapter. This shows differences in the design of each measure. Reading age is approximately FKG + 5. Range is the possible mean score range of values from floor to ceiling for a group of patients. Direction shows that a high score for MYCaW is bad, but good for PSO.

Conclusions

Individualised measures allow patients to say what is most important for them, rather than treating all patients the same. This is a core principle of patient-centred care. Individualised measures are complementary to generic and condition-specific measures.

Table 14.1 Comparison of measures showing: number of items, number of response options, recall period, word count, Flesch-Kincaid Grade (FKG) readability measure, range and direction

Measure	Items	Options	Recall	Words	FKG	Range	Direction
MYCaW	3	7	Now	181	3.4	0 to 6	Negative
PSO	2	4	Now	65	1.2	0 to 100	Positive

References

1. Porter I, Gonçalves-Bradley D, Ricci-Cabello I, et al. Framework and guidance for implementing patient-reported outcomes in clinical practice: evidence, challenges and opportunities. J Comp Effect Res. 2016;5(5):507–19.
2. Dijkers MP. Individualization in quality of life measurement: instruments and approaches. Arch Phys Med Rehabil. 2003;84:S3–14.
3. Browne JP, O'Boyle CA, McGee HM, et al. Individual quality of life in the healthy elderly. Qual Life Res. 1994;3:235–44.
4. Ruta DA, Garratt AM, Leng M, et al. A new approach to the measurement of quality of life: the patient generated index. Med Care. 1994;32(11):1109–26.
5. Paterson C. Measuring outcomes in primary care: a patient generated measure, MYMOP, compared with the SF-36 health survey. BMJ. 1996;312(7037):1016–20.
6. Paterson C, Thomas K, Manasse A, et al. Measure Yourself Concerns and Wellbeing (MYCaW): an individualised questionnaire for evaluating outcome in cancer support care that includes complementary therapies. Complem Ther Med. 2007;15(1):38–45.
7. Jolliffe R, Seers H, Jackson S, et al. The responsiveness, content validity, and convergent validity of the measure yourself concerns and wellbeing (MYCaW) patient-reported outcome measure. Integr Cancer Ther. 2015;14(1):26–34.
8. Jolliffe R, Collaco N, Seers H, et al. Development of measure yourself concerns and wellbeing for informal caregivers of people with cancer—a multicentred study. Support Care Cancer. 2019;27(5):1901–9.
9. Benson T. Person-specific outcome measure (PSO) for use in primary and community care. BMJ Open Qual. 2021;10:e001379.
10. Benson T. Measure what we want: a taxonomy of short generic patient and staff-reported outcome and experience measures (PROMs and PREMs). BMJ Open Qual. 2020;9:e000789.
11. Benson T, Sizmur S, Whatling J, et al. Evaluation of a new short generic measure of health status: howRu. J Innov Health Inform. 2010;18:89–101.
12. Benson T, Sladen J, Liles A, et al. Personal Wellbeing Score (PWS)—a short version of ONS4: development and validation in social prescribing. BMJ Open Quality. 2019;8(2):e000394.
13. Benson T, Potts HW, Bark P, et al. Development and initial testing of a Health Confidence Score (HCS). BMJ Open Qual. 2019;8(2):e000411.

How People Live 15

Social Determinants of Health

Social determinants of health (SDoH) include all non-medical factors that influence health outcomes such as income, education, employment, food, housing, environment, child development, discrimination, and war. Some 80% of our health depends on these factors, while only 20% depends on the health care we receive. Health inequity and social injustice are killing people on a grand scale [1].

There is plenty of evidence that SDoH and health inequalities are the most important factors affecting health outcomes. They are more important than health services or lifestyle choices in impacting health. For example, people born in developed counties have life expectancy 19 years longer than those born in low development countries. In one London borough there is a 16 year difference between people living in the least and most deprived parts. People with low education have twice as much poor health as do university-educated people. The incidence and mortality rates of people catching COVID-19 living in deprived areas is double that of the least deprived areas [2, 3].

Health Index for England

Most SDoH measures focus on how and where people live and use existing data, which was collected for other reasons. These measures are aimed primarily at informing national and regional policy makers. For example, the Health Index for England developed by the Office of National Statistics (ONS) has a single summary score and three broad domains [4]:

- *Healthy people*, which focuses on health outcomes. This includes mortality, physical health conditions, disability and frailty, personal wellbeing and mental health.

- *Healthy lives*, which captures health-related behavior. This includes physiological and behavioral risk factors, unemployment, working conditions, children's risk factors and education, and protective measures.
- *Healthy places*, which captures wider determinants of health and environmental factors. This includes green space, local environment, housing, medical and leisure services, and crime rates.

Each domain has subdomains and the whole index uses 58 indicators, chosen in part because they were available at the time the index was created [5]. The Health Index for England allows policy makers to compare local authority areas at national, regional and district levels.

Social Determinants Measure

SDoH refers to the conditions in which people are born, grow, live, work and age [6]. We also wanted to capture individuals' own perception of their situation. This is in line with the importance of self-perceived social standing or status, as illustrated by Oscar-winning actors living four years longer than the nominated actors who did not win Oscars [7].

Working with social prescribing projects in the South of England, we found that results in different areas were impacted by the underlying SDoH of those being helped. Even areas with high mean SDoH scores contain individuals with low SDoH.

In about 2016, we investigated the possibility of developing a measure of SDoH for individuals. We focused on individuals because it was often not meaningful to compare the health outcomes of individuals with good SDoH with those with poor SDoH.

Various forms have been piloted, although the results are not directly comparable with that shown here. As usual, our starting point was to review the literature and to synthesize a few key factors, which could be expressed in simple questions that people could answer consistently.

We identified the following factors and associated items:

- Education—*I have had a good education*. This covers all types of education and the conditions in which people are born and grow. In the USA there is a large difference in mortality rates between white people who have and do not have a degree [8].
- Control—*I feel in control of what I do*. This focuses on the concept of self-efficacy and social status within the community.
- Housing/environment—*I am happy about where I live*. This covers housing, environment as well as how people live and age.
- Poverty—*I have enough money to cope*. This covers how people live and age.

Social Determinants

Thinking about how you live

	Strongly agree	Agree	Disagree	Strongly disagree
I have had a good education	😀	🙂	🙁	☹️
I feel in control of what I do	😀	🙂	🙁	☹️
I am happy about where I live	😀	🙂	🙁	☹️
I have enough money to cope	😀	🙂	🙁	☹️

Fig. 15.1 Social determinants of health measure for individuals

Following the pattern used in other measures, we use four response options: *Strongly agree, Agree, Disagree* and *Strongly disagree* with optional coloured emojis. For individuals, items are scored 3, 2, 1 and 0 respectively and a summary score is calculated as a sum of the item scores, giving a scale from 12 to 0. For cohorts, mean scores are used for both items and the summary score, on a scale from 100 (ceiling) to 0 (floor). A high score is good, and a low score is bad.

The resulting format is shown in Fig. 15.1.

This short generic measure of individual SDoH is designed for use in clinical situations, along-side other measures in the R-Outcomes family of patient-reported outcome and experience measures (PROMs and PREMs).

The measure shown here differs from that previously published [9]. The item *I feel in control of what I do* has been changed, following consultations and discussions, from *I am valued for what I do*. Both phrases address the concept of social standing or status but being in control is aligned more with ideas of locus of control and self-efficacy. The original phrase had a greater overlap with ideas of fulfilment and eudemonia, which are captured in the Personal Wellbeing Score (PWS) by *What I do in my life is worthwhile* [10].

Two response options have also been changed from *Neutral* and *Disagree* to *Disagree* and *Strongly disagree* respectively, with corresponding changes to emojis, reflecting the high level of inequality in many societies.

This SDoH measure is mainly designed to collect baseline data when a patient is referred to a service. Most clinical interventions do not impact SDoH directly, so this is not a conventional PROM, which measures the effectiveness of interventions, nor a conventional PREM, which measures service satisfaction. Rather, it is a way of quantifying the context in which an intervention takes place.

However, some interventions, such as social prescribing, may be targeted directly at SDoH, by signposting patients to detailed advice about life-long learning (education), counselling (control), housing services (housing/environment) or benefits (poverty) [11].

Loneliness and Social Contact

Loneliness is defined as the *unpleasant experience that occurs when a person's network of social relations is deficient in some important way, either quantitatively or qualitatively* [12]. It affects all ages and has sub-categories of social, emotional, and existential loneliness [13]. *Social loneliness* occurs when the quantity and quality of social relationships does not match those we want. *Emotional loneliness* is the absence of meaningful relationships. *Existential loneliness* is less related to the specifics of relationships but is focused on a more global evaluation of disconnection from others and the wider world.

Here, we treat loneliness and the perception of lack of social contact as synonymous. Loneliness is a negative term while social contact is more positive. Social isolation is different. Some socially isolated people do not feel the lack of social contact or feel lonely, although others do.

Loneliness impacts other measures of health and wellbeing. Mortality rates are more than 25% higher for lonely people [14, 15]. During the COVID-19 pandemic awareness of the extent and impact of loneliness across the whole population increased, although the risk factors did not change [16, 17].

Loneliness Measures

Loneliness measures may be direct, or indirect. Direct measures of loneliness ask specifically about loneliness, usually with a single item.

Indirect measures cover multiple aspects of the concept of loneliness, and many avoid using the terms *lonely* or *loneliness*. They can indicate what might be done to reduce loneliness.

Indirect loneliness measures include: the UCLA loneliness scale with 3 items having 3 options each [18]; the De Jong Gierfeld Loneliness scale with 6 items having 3 options each and distinguishes between emotional and social aspects [19]; and the Campaign to End Loneliness scale with 3 items having 5 options each [20].

In 2018, the UK Department for Digital, Culture and Sport issued a major report on loneliness, setting out a national vision to end loneliness within our lifetimes. It included a commitment to produce a new national measure of loneliness [15]. The Office of National Statistics (ONS) issued recommendations on how to measure loneliness in large-scale national surveys [21]. A central principle was to re-use existing measures, not to develop new ones [22]. In 2020, the Government Statistical Service issued a GSS Loneliness Harmonised Standard, based on work by ONS. This is based on the UCLA loneliness scale plus a direct measure with 5 options [23].

Social Contact

Customers, who were using R-Outcomes measures in social prescribing, asked us to develop a compatible measure of social contact/loneliness. Here, we describe both the R-Outcomes Social Contact and Loneliness measures [24]. At the end of this chapter, we compare these with other widely-used measures for number if items, options, length, readability, range, etc.

Our work on Social Contact and Loneliness started in about 2016. The Social Contact measure is described first, followed by the Loneliness measure. We had previously developed several PROMs covering health status (Chap. 11), personal well-being (Chap. 12), health confidence (Chap. 13), and experience (Chap. 10). These measures share a common look and feel, based the following common principles and format:

- Applicable to all people irrespective of their age, gender, health conditions or any other factors.
- Short, with a low reading age.
- Four items per measure (although this is not essential). Positive wording.
- Four options for each item, listed from good to bad. Optional use of colour and emojis for each option to indicate good (green smile), bad (sad red) and so on.
- Cover multiple aspects of the concept recognised in the literature.
- Generate a single summary score for use alongside item scores.
- Mean item and summary scores for a group are reported using a 0–100 scale, where a high mean score is always better than a low mean score. This means that a before and after improvement is always a positive number.

No existing measures met these criteria, so we developed a new measure. We studied the literature to identify the most important aspects of the subject identified by academic research and held informal focus groups with actual and potential customers, to understand user needs. The measure evolved over about four years.

In addition to the criteria set out above, we aimed to cover both emotional loneliness and social loneliness, use positive wording, and focus on what prevents or ameliorates loneliness. We also wanted to avoid using a recall period, such as a week or a month or ask about frequency, because human memory is fallible and recall periods are a source of unreliability [25]. For this reason we ask about people's perception, using options: Strongly agree, Agree, Neutral and Disagree.

We settled on four items:

1. *I have people to talk to*—this covers peoples' social need for companionship.
2. *I have someone I can confide in*—this covers our need for close emotional contacts.
3. *I have people who will help me*—this covers our need for practical social relationships when needed.
4. *I do things with others*—this covers our need to feel included, or not feeling left out.

The final social contact measure is shown in Fig. 15.2.

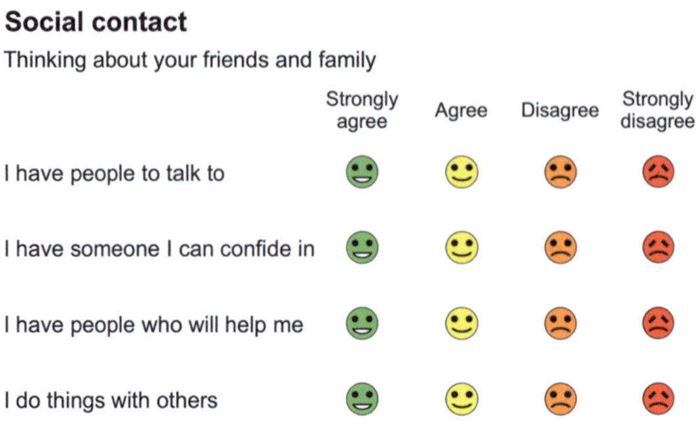

Social contact

Thinking about your friends and family

	Strongly agree	Agree	Disagree	Strongly disagree
I have people to talk to	😀	🙂	☹️	😞
I have someone I can confide in	😀	🙂	☹️	😞
I have people who will help me	😀	🙂	☹️	😞
I do things with others	😀	🙂	☹️	😞

Fig. 15.2 Social contact measure

Loneliness

When the ONS issued early versions of what became GSS Loneliness Harmonised Standard (referred to as GSS standard) [21, 23], we set out to incorporate these into a format compatible with the criteria stated above. We aimed to avoid three features we thought to be undesirable: (1) three items with three options each and one item with five options, (2) different methods of scoring different items, and (3) improvements (reduced loneliness) shown as negative numbers.

In the GSS standard, the first three questions use options: *hardly ever or never* (which is scored as one), *some of the time* (2), and *often* (3). These three item scores are summed to create a total, with a range from 3 to 9. There is no accepted level for which to consider a person *lonely*. However, it is useful to observe changes in average score over time or compare the average scores of different groups.

The fourth question in the GSS standard may be reported by percentage of respondents selecting each response option. ONS suggests defining levels of loneliness in a population as the proportion of people reporting *often or always* feeling lonely.

We modified the GSS standard proposals in a way similar to what we did with ONS4 personal well-being questions (see Chap. 12). Figure 15.3 shows the resulting Loneliness measure. This meets the criteria listed above, apart from positive wording. The biggest change from the GSS standard is the use of four consistent simplified options for each item, from worst to best (*Often*, *Sometimes*, *Occasionally* and *Hardly ever*).

Loneliness

How often do you …

	Hardly ever	Occasionally	Sometimes	Often
Have no-one to talk to?	😀	🙂	😕	☹️
Feel left out?	😀	🙂	😕	☹️
Feel alone?	😀	🙂	😕	☹️
Feel lonely	😀	🙂	😕	☹️

Fig. 15.3 R-Outcomes loneliness measure

Case Study—Social Contact

A convenience sample of results was analysed from Tri Locality Care Ltd, which provides social prescribing and other services for patients in an area north-west of Southampton, England, which is not deprived. Detailed information is available in the full paper [24].

This study focuses on the Social contact measure, but also uses measures for social determinants of health (SDoH) (two items), health status, health confidence, personal wellbeing (two items), and patient experience, which are described elsewhere in this book.

Patients were asked by a staff member to complete surveys at the time of their first visit (n = 411) and last scheduled visit (typically 6–8 weeks later, n = 322). Patients entered the data directly into a tablet or reported to a staff member who performed data entry. During the COVID-19 pandemic face-to-face visits were replaced by telephone calls. About 60% of respondents were over 80 years old.

Table 15.1 shows the mean score for each group (All, Before and After) for social contact items, two social determinants of health (SDoH) items (*I am happy about where I live* and *I have enough money to cope*), and other measures summary scores. It also shows the difference between Before (B) and After (A) scores (A − B), and the probability that changes could be by chance (p-values); all are statistically significant ($p < 0.05$).

The four items in the Social contact measure address different aspects of loneliness and the mean scores differ a lot. It helps to report the mean scores for each item individually as well as the summary score. The highest mean score (76.1) is for *I have people who will help* me while the lowest mean score (46.8) is for *I do things with others*. This may reflect good neighbour relations in the first instance and patients' disability and the impact of the COVID pandemic in the second. Low

Table 15.1 Social contact item and summary scores for All, Before (n = 411), After (n = 322), difference (A − B) and p-values (t-test)

Measure	All	Before (B)	After (A)	Diff (A − B)	p
Social contact items					
I have people to talk to	58.5	56.0	61.8	5.8	0.008
I have someone I can confide in	70.1	66.8	74.2	7.4	<0.001
I have people who will help me	76.1	73.2	79.8	6.6	<0.001
I do things with others	46.8	43.7	50.8	6.9	<0.001
Summary scores					
Social contact summary score	62.9	59.9	66.7	6.8	<0.001
Social determinants (2 items)	67.9	65.6	70.9	5.3	0.011
Health status (*howRu*)	56.0	52.9	60.1	7.2	<0.001
Health confidence (HCS)	64.5	60.7	69.5	8.8	<0.001
Personal wellbeing (2 items)	48.2	43.2	54.8	11.6	<0.001
Patient experience (*howRwe*)	81.3	75.1	89.5	14.4	<0.001

scores on any items may prompt a member of staff to consider if and how they can alleviate the problems identified.

The lowest mean summary score is for the two personal well-being items (48.2) is; these items are: *I was happy yesterday* and *I was NOT anxious yesterday*.

The highest mean summary score is for Patient experience (81.3). Personal wellbeing and Patient experience showed the greatest improvement (11.6 and 14.4 respectively). Both respond well to the support offered by social prescribing service.

The smallest mean changes are for *I have people to talk to* and the two SDoH items (*I am happy about where I live* and *I have enough money to cope*). These are harder to change.

Table 15.2 shows the inter-item correlation matrix. In this population the item *I do things with others* has a lower inter-item correlation than the other items. This may be due to multiple factors: most respondents are over 80 years old with disability, many have lost their partners and some data was collected during the COVID pandemic. Cronbach's $\alpha = 0.76$, which taken together with the inter-item correlation matrix suggests that it is appropriate to have a summary score as well as the four items.

Table 15.3 shows correlations between different types of measure. The highest correlation is between personal wellbeing (PWS) and health status (*howRu*), which includes an item on well-being ($r = 0.51$). Social contact, Personal wellbeing (PWS) and social determinants (SDoH) are also moderately correlated. The lowest is between loneliness and patient experience ($r = 0.25$). People with higher health confidence and higher SDOH tend to report better patient experience. All correlations are significant.

Case Study—Social Contact

Table 15.2 Inter-item Pearson correlation matrix (all data)

Item text	I have people to talk to	I have someone I can confide in	I have people who will help me
I have people to talk to	–		
I have someone I can confide in	0.56	–	
I have people who will help me	0.41	0.69	–
I do things with others	0.38	0.32	0.35

Table 15.3 Pearson correlation matrix for each measure's summary scores (all data). All correlations are significant ($p < 0.001$)

Variable	Social contact	Health status (*howRu*)	Health confidence (HCS)	Personal wellbeing (PWS)*	Social determinants (SDoH)*
Social contact	–				
Health status (*howRu*)	0.32	–			
Health confidence (HCS)	0.30	0.38	–		
Personal wellbeing (PWS)*	0.49	0.51	0.24	–	
Social determinants (SDoH)*	0.47	0.37	0.30	0.48	–
Patient experience (*howRwe*)	0.25	0.28	0.40	0.26	0.36

* Only two items asked

Exploratory factor analysis showed that each measure addresses a different concept.

The results are consistent with expectations, providing strong evidence of construct validation.

- Social contact improves following social prescribing intervention—before 60, after 67 ($p < 0.001$) [26].
- Social contact is lower in women than men—women 61, men 65, ($p < 0.01$) [26].
- Perceived social contact scores are lower in younger people—ANOVA by age group ($p < 0.001$) [27].

- Social contact is moderately correlated with personal well-being (PWS) ($r = 0.49$) [28].
- Social contact is moderately correlated with social determinants of health (SDoH) ($r = 0.47$) [29].
- Social contact is moderately correlated with health status (*howRu*) ($r = 0.32$) [30].
- Social contact is moderately correlated with health confidence (HCS) ($r = 0.30$) [31].
- Social contact is weakly correlated with patient experience (*howRwe*) ($r = 0.25$) [32].

Discussion

These measures are designed for use in local projects, such as in social prescribing, where respondent burden is important and other domains need to be measured as well as social contact. They combine well with other measures, which can be picked and mixed to meet local needs. For all measures a high score is good, so any improvement is shown as a positive number and deterioration as a negative number.

Completing PROMs may help patients think about themselves in ways that are beneficial. This information can also help clinicians build relationships with patients based on better understanding of how they live [33].

We do not know whether any improvements in social contact/loneliness or other measures will be sustained. However, we can say that patients report better social contact scores and other patient-reported measures after social prescribing help than before. This study adds to the evidence that social prescribing delivers benefits across multiple dimensions.

The largest differences between before and after ratings are in patient experience and personal wellbeing. These may have improved because social prescribing link workers have more time than GPs and other clinical staff to listen to patients' problems, help and explain issues. Other domains, which are harder for social prescribing interventions to change for most people, show smaller improvements. These include housing and poverty (SDoH) and underlying health conditions (health status). Social contact falls somewhere in the middle.

Length and Readability

Table 15.4 compares the word count, Flesch-Kincaid readability grade (FKG), the number of positively and negatively worded items and the range of scores possible for a group of people for the measures mentioned in this chapter. This shows differences in the design of each measure.

Word count and FKG include the items, preamble, and options, but not the title or any copyright notices. FKG was calculated using the *readingformulas.com* web site. Reading age is approximately FKG + 5. Range is the possible score range of values from floor to ceiling. Score range differs considerably. For groups of people

Table 15.4 Comparison of loneliness and SDoH measures

Variable	Items	Options	Words	FKG	Wording	Range	Improve
Social contact	4	4	36	3.7	Positive	0 to 100	Positive
Loneliness	4	4	21	4.8	Negative	0 to 100	Positive
Social determinants (SDoH)	4	4	38	3.4	Positive	0 to 100	Positive
GSS loneliness	4	3 with 3 1 with 5	75	5.5	Negative	3–9% in top 2	Negative
De Jong Gierveld-6	6	3	78	3.2	3 Positive 3 Negative	0 to 6	Negative
Campaign to end loneliness	3	5	67	7.0	Positive	0 to 12	Negative

the mean R-Outcomes scores are reported on a 0–100 scale for each item and the summary score, where a high score is good. Improvement is always a positive number.

References

1. Commission on Social Determinants of Health. Closing the gap in a generation: health equity through action on the social determinants of health. Geneva: World Health Organization; 2008.
2. WHO. Social determinants of health. Health topic. https://www.who.int/health-topics/social-determinants-of-health. Accessed 7 Oct 2021.
3. Marmot M, Allen J. COVID-19: exposing and amplifying inequalities. J Epidemiol Community Health. 2020; 74(9):681–2.
4. Pearson-Stuttard J, Davis S. The health index for England. Lancet. 2021; 397:665.
5. Ceely G. Developing the health index for England: 2015 to 2018. ONS; 2020. https://www.ons.gov.uk/peoplepopulationandcommunity/healthandsocialcare/healthandwellbeing/articles/developingthehealthindexforengland/2015to2018. Accessed 7 Mar 2021.
6. Marmot M. The health gap: the challenge of an unequal world. London: Bloomsbury; 2015.
7. Marmot M. Status syndrome: how your social standing directly affects your health and life expectancy. London: Bloomsbury; 2004.
8. Case A, Deaton A. Deaths of despair and the future of capitalism. Princeton NJ: Princeton University Press; 2020.
9. Benson T. Measure what we want: a taxonomy of short generic person-reported outcome and experience measures (PROMs and PREMs). BMJ Open Qual. 2020; 9:e000789.
10. Benson T, Sladen J, Liles A, et al. Personal Wellbeing Score (PWS)-a short version of ONS4: development and validation in social prescribing. BMJ Open Qual. 2019; 8:e000394.
11. Jani A, Liyanage H, Hoang U, et al. Use and impact of social prescribing: a mixed-methods feasibility study protocol. BMJ Open 2020; 10:e037681.
12. Perlman D, Peplau L. Toward a social psychology of loneliness. In: Gilmour R, Duck S editors. Personal relationships: 3. Relationships in disorder. London UK: Academic Press; 1981. p. 31–56.
13. Mansfield L, Daykin N, Meads C, et al. A conceptual review of loneliness across the adult life course (16+ years): synthesis of qualitative studies. London UK: What Works Wellbeing; 2019.

14. Holt-Lunstad J, Smith T, Baker M, Harris T, Stephenson D. Loneliness and social isolation as risk factors for mortality: a meta-analytic review. Perspect Psychol Sci. 2015; 10:227–37.
15. HM Government. A connected society: a strategy for tackling loneliness—laying the foundations for change. London UK: Department for Digital, Culture, Media and Sport; 2018.
16. Groarke J, Berry E, Graham-Wisener L, et al. Loneliness in the UK during the COVID-19 pandemic: cross-sectional results from the COVID-19 psychological wellbeing study. PLoS ONE 2020; 15(9):e0239698.
17. Rees E, Large R. Coronavirus and loneliness, Great Britain: 3 April to 3 May 2020: analysis of loneliness in Great Britain during the coronavirus (COVID-19) pandemic from the opinions and lifestyle survey. Office of National Statistics 2020. https://www.ons.gov.uk/peoplepopulationandcommunity/wellbeing/bulletins/coronavirusandlonelinessgreatbritain/3aprilto3may2020. Accessed 9 Nov 2020.
18. Hughes ME, Waite LJ, Hawkley LC, Cacioppo JT. A short scale for measuring loneliness in large surveys: results from two population-based studies. Res Ageing. 2004; 26(6):655–72.
19. De Jong GJ, van Tilburg T. 6-Item scale for overall, emotional, and social loneliness: confirmatory tests on survey data. Res Ageing. 2006; 28(5):582–98.
20. Goodman A. Measuring your impact on loneliness in later life. London UK: Campaign to End Loneliness; 2015.
21. Snape D, Martin G. Measuring loneliness: guidance for use of the national indicators on surveys. ONS; 2018.
22. Snape D, Pyle E. Mapping the loneliness measurement landscape. ONS; 2018.
23. Nickson S. Loneliness harmonised standard. London: Government Statistical Service;2020. https://gss.civilservice.gov.uk/policy-store/loneliness-indicators/. Accessed 31 Mar 2021.
24. Benson T, Seers H, Webb N, McMahon P. Development of social contact and loneliness measures with validation in social prescribing. BMJ Open Qual. 2021; 10(2):e001306.
25. Condon DM, Chapman R, Shaunfield S, et al. Does recall period matter? Comparing PROMIS® physical function with no recall, 24-hr recall, and 7-day recall. Qual Life Res. 2020; 29(3):745–53.
26. Foster A, Thompson J, Holding E, et al. Impact of social prescribing to address loneliness: a mixed methods evaluation of a national social prescribing programme. Health Soc Care Community. 2020; 00:1–11.
27. Dahlberg L, Agahi N, Lennartsson C. Lonelier than ever? Loneliness of older people over two decades. Arch Gerontol Geriatr. 2018; 75:96–103.
28. VanderWeele T, Hawkley L, Cacioppo J. On the reciprocal association between loneliness and subjective well-being. Am J Epidemiol. 2012; 176(9):77–84.
29. Scharf T, De Jong GJ. Loneliness in urban neighbourhoods: an Anglo-Dutch comparison. Eur J Ageing. 2008; 5(2):103–16.
30. Henriksen J, Larsen E, Mattisson C, Andersson N. Loneliness, health and mortality. Epidemiol Psychiatr Sci. 2019; 28(2):234–9.
31. Suanet B, van Tilburg TG. Loneliness declines across birth cohorts: the impact of mastery and self-efficacy. Psychol Aging. 2019; 34(8):1134–43.
32. Aoki T, Yamamoto Y, Ikenoue T, et al. Social isolation and patient experience in older adults. Ann Fam Med. 2018; 16(5):393–8.
33. Hamilton-West K, Milne A, Hotham S. New horizons in supporting older people's health and wellbeing: is social prescribing a way forward? Age Ageing. 2020; 49(3):319–26.

Innovation Evaluation 16

Innovation

This chapter outlines uses of PROMs and PREMs in evaluation of health innovations. These fall slightly outside the usual focus of PROMs and PREMs, but innovation impact evaluation makes extensive use of surveys as well as qualitative research. Innovation spread is vital for the future improvement of health care and many innovations are designed to improve outcomes or experience directly or indirectly.

The health services can sometimes adopt new innovations remarkably quickly, such as during the COVID pandemic, but other innovations take a very long time. To take one example, laparoscopic surgery was used routinely by gynaecologists for two decades before it was adopted by general surgeons [1]. Stop-gap processes are often used decades after their original designers thought they would be replaced.

Innovation may be defined ias as a product such as a new idea, method or device; as a process, such as the introduction and adoption of new ideas, discoveries and inventions; or as an outcome, such as significant measurable change.

Most products do not even get to the market unless they offer some benefit. Often a product performs well where it was developed but not nearly as well in other places. Our focus here is on innovation spread and process. Outcomes can be measured using measures described elsewhere in this book.

In recent years, a lot of effort has been devoted to understanding better how and why healthcare innovations do or do not spread. The focus is often the innovation itself (technology), but other factors are often more critical in determining success or failure [2]. Healthcare innovation spread is seldom a simple linear process. It involves a complex adaptive system where unpredictability and uncertainty are the norm [3].

The NASSS framework (described in Chap. 5) helps explain many of the reasons for non-adoption, abandonment and challenges to scale-up, spread and sustainability of patient-facing health and care technologies [4].

NASS has seven dimensions:

1. The clinical condition(s) being treated
2. Technologies used
3. The value proposition
4. The adopter system (staff, patients, carers)
5. The organisations involved and their culture
6. The wider context including government and regulation
7. Interaction between domains and adaptation over time.

Issues in any one dimension can cause an innovation to fail; multiple issues, in more than one dimension, are a recipe for failure.

Measures

The measures described in this chapter were prompted by working on the evaluation of digital innovations and new care models in health and care services. We sought short simple generic survey tools to meet our evaluation needs but could not find what we needed. As a result, we developed a set of related measures, after reviewing the innovation literature and based on our experience in developing person-reported outcome measures (PROMs) and person-reported experience measures (PREMs).

The measures described here are:

- **Innovation readiness** helps show where users and organisations lie on the innovativeness spectrum. It is based on Rogers' categories of innovator, early adopter, early majority, late majority and laggard [5].
- **Digital confidence** helps find out about patients' digital literacy and confidence to use digital products.
- **Innovation process** rates the process of adoption, before, during and after implementation. It is based on May's Normalisation Process Theory (NPT) [6].
- **User satisfaction** is the user's assessment of a specific digital product, as a combination of customer satisfaction and user experience (in its widest sense).
- **Behaviour change** helps identify factors, such as capability, opportunity and motivation that stop us doing what is being proposed. It is based on Michie's COM-B model [7].
- **Training** is based on Kirkpatrick's four levels—reaction, learning, behaviour and results [8].
- **Digital competence** is staff's capability to adopt, use and spread digital healthcare technologies effectively.
- **Product confidence** is staff's confidence to use a product well.

These measures share the same look and feel as other short generic PROMs and PREMs described in this book. Design criteria include being clear, brief, suitable for frequent use, multi-modal (suitable for use with multiple data collection modalities including smart-phones), responsive, good psychometric properties and easily understood scores and data visualisation. Scores generated are easy to interpret and act on by all stakeholders, as well as being comparable for benchmarking.

Each measure is short with a low reading age and generic, applicable for any condition in any setting. Each has four items, although exceptions are allowed, with four response options each. Options are labelled, colour-coded and use emoji. For scoring, each option is allocated a score on a 0–3 scale, where: Strongly agree = 3, Agree = 2, Neutral = 1, and Disagree = 0. A higher score is always better.

A summary score for a group of four items is calculated by adding the scores for each item, giving a 13-point scale with a range from 0 (4× disagree) to 12 (4× strongly agree). When reporting results for a cohort, the mean scores for items and the summary scores are transformed linearly to a scale from 0 to 100, where 0 indicates that all respondents chose the lowest score (the floor) and 100 that all chose the highest (the ceiling). The 0–100 scale is familiar and enables comparison of item and summary mean scores on the same scale.

Each measure was developed in a similar way. We identified the need for a measure, reviewed the literature, consulted with colleagues and users, designed prototypes and the measures evolved through a series of iterations with input from users and colleagues over several years.

Innovation Readiness

The concept of innovation readiness or innovativeness is based on Rogers' classic work on innovation diffusion [5]. Innovativeness is the degree to which an individual or organisation is earlier in adopting new ideas than other members of the system. At the individual level, members of a social system may be classified into adopter categories on the basis of their innovativeness. The numbers in parenthesis show the expected percentage of a population found in each group, based on normal distribution.

1. Innovators, who are often mavericks who like to think outside the box (2%)
2. Early adopters, typically visionary and locally respected (14%)
3. Early majority, who are pragmatic and deliberate before choosing (34%)
4. Late majority, who are generally conservative and sceptical of change (34%)
5. Laggards, traditionalists who dislike almost all change (16%).

For individuals, the innovation-decision process is an information-seeking and information-processing activity to understand the advantages and disadvantages of the innovation. It starts once a need has been recognised and includes: knowledge acquisition, persuasion of decision makers, the decision to adopt or reject, implementation processes, and finally, confirmation, evaluation and promotion.

The rate of adoption is measured by how long it takes for a certain proportion of the members of a system to use the innovation. Innovators and early adopters have shorter innovation-decision periods than late adopters and laggards. Aspects of innovations that help explain different rates of adoption include:1. relative advantage—better than what it replaces; 2. compatibility—consistent with values, needs and past experience; 3. complexity—ease of understanding; 4. trialability—easy to test or pilot; 5. observability or visibility; 6. adaptability to local context; and 7. evidence base.

Spread covers both diffusion and dissemination of innovations, which are complementary concepts. Diffusion is horizontal, usually unplanned and subjective, through peer networks. Dissemination is vertical, planned, and targeted top-down from the centre, usually based on experts' recommendations.

Within organisations, the innovation process has five stages:

1. Agenda—identify a need
2. Match—fit a solution with a problem
3. Redefine/restructure—adapt the organisation and/or the innovation to each other
4. Clarify—the meaning of the innovation becomes clearer to the organisation's members
5. Routinise—the innovation is widely used and sustainable. It becomes the way we do things here.

For individuals, each adopter type on the innovativeness spectrum has characteristic differences in terms of socio-economic status, personality values and communication behaviour. Attributes of early adopters and innovators are optimism, openness and being well informed about new ideas. To capture this, we have:

- *New ideas are needed* (openness)
- *I keep up to date with new ideas* (well-informed).

The early majority are pragmatists, who place great emphasis on referrals and the opinions of other users. They are most comfortable when they pick the market leader in any field. The late majority are conservatives, who are happy to wait until costs have fallen as low as they will ever be. Finally, laggards only change their ways if there is no alternative.

Organisations and their leaders also fall on the innovativeness spectrum, with some being innovators and early adopters and others are pragmatic, conservative or resist all change for as long as possible. All innovation involves adaptive change

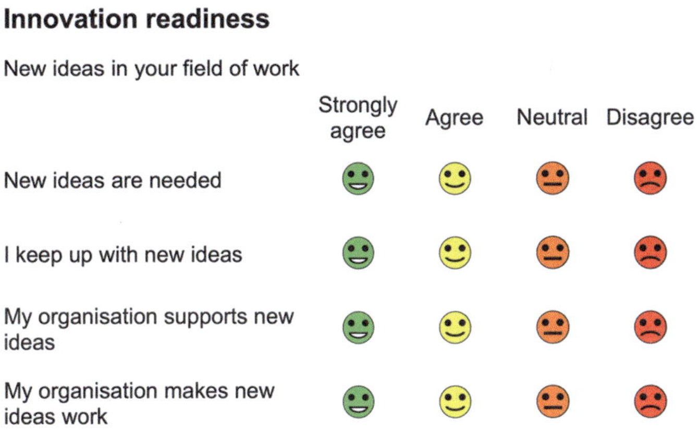

Innovation readiness

New ideas in your field of work

	Strongly agree	Agree	Neutral	Disagree
New ideas are needed	😀	🙂	😐	☹️
I keep up with new ideas	😀	🙂	😐	☹️
My organisation supports new ideas	😀	🙂	😐	☹️
My organisation makes new ideas work	😀	🙂	😐	☹️

Fig. 16.1 Innovation readiness measure

and puts pressure on staff at all levels [9]. Attributes for success include a culture of receptiveness to new ideas and the organisation's capability, capacity and perseverance to make changes work. To capture this we use:

- *My organisation supports new ideas* (receptiveness)
- *My organisation makes new ideas work* (capability).

The Innovation Readiness measure (Fig. 16.1) is mainly used by staff working in organisations.

Digital Confidence

The digital divide is a problem especially in health and social care, where many patients are old, infirm and suffer from cognitive challenges such as dementia [10].

Digital literacy is the knowledge, skills, and behaviours used in a broad range of digital devices such as smartphones, tablets, laptops, and desktop PCs. It includes computer, network, information and social media literacy, and computer self-efficacy [11].

The Computer Self-Efficacy measure focuses on a computer software package designed to make your life easier that you have not used before [12]. It has 10 question items, rated using a 10-point scale and is focused on computer systems used at work.

Digital confidence

Digital devices include computers, tablets and smartphones

	Strongly agree	Agree	Neutral	Disagree
I use a digital device frequently	😀	🙂	😐	☹️
Most of my friends use digital devices	😀	🙂	😐	☹️
I can usually get help if stuck	😀	🙂	😐	☹️
I feel confident using most digital devices	😀	🙂	😐	☹️

Fig. 16.2 Digital confidence score

Our focus was on older patients' confidence to use digital devices in their own time. The purpose of a digital confidence score is to self-rate people for their level of digital self-efficacy, so that people who need more help can get it.

The Digital Confidence Score (Fig. 16.2) has 4 items:

- Familiarity—*I use a digital device frequently.*
- Social pressure—*Most of my friends use digital devices.*
- Support—*I can usually get help if I am stuck.*
- Digital self-efficacy—*I feel confident using most digital devices.*

The Digital Competence score, described below, has a similar name but has some differences and is aimed at staff who use already computers in their day-to-day work.

Innovation Process

Normalisation Process Theory (NPT) was developed to help understand the dynamics of implementation of complex interventions in health care [7]. It helps explain how new methods and processes become routinely embedded in their contexts, based on four mechanisms:

- Coherence of the original vision
- Cognitive participation and planning
- Collective action to make it work
- Reflexive monitoring to make it better.

NPT focuses on the work that people do at each stage. Traditionally, NPT has been used by trained interviewers with staff collecting qualitative (narrative) answers to 16 questions (NoMAD) [13].

Working with NPT practitioners, we looked at the feasibility of creating a staff-reported module related to NPT to help evaluate specific innovations. This is shown in Fig. 16.3. This uses an agree/disagree structure, with four items to be asked of staff about their experience in working on a specific project:

- Coherence—*Is the original vision being followed?*
- Cognitive participation—*Did staff plan in advance how to make it work?*
- Collective action—*Do staff work together to make it work?*
- Reflexive monitoring—*Do staff reflect on how best to improve it?*

Product Satisfaction

Evaluators need a tool to measure user's experience of a digital tool or product, which can be used, either soon after starting to use a product or after several months of use. The scope should cover all software products, not only apps used on mobile devices. Applications have many purposes, and a generic rating tool needs to cope with a very wide range of use cases. Some such tools exist; one is the Mobile App Rating Scale (MARS), although it is not designed for end users. MARS has over 2,000 words and has a reading age of 14 [14].

The *Product satisfaction* measure is a short generic questionnaire to allow end users to rate their perceptions of a specific software application or product (Fig. 16.4).

Innovation process

Thinking about this project

	Strongly agree	Agree	Neutral	Disagree
Is the original vision is being followed?	😀	🙂	😐	☹️
Did staff plan in advance how to make it work?	😀	🙂	😐	☹️
Do staff work together to make it work?	😀	🙂	😐	☹️
Do staff reflect on how best to improve it?	😀	🙂	😐	☹️

Fig. 16.3 Innovation process measure

Product satisfaction

What do you think of this product?

	Strongly agree	Agree	Neutral	Disagree
It helps me do what I want	😀	🙂	😐	☹️
It is easy to use	😀	🙂	😐	☹️
I can get help if I need it	😀	🙂	😐	☹️
I am satisfied with this product	😀	🙂	😐	☹️

Fig. 16.4 User satisfaction measure

The four items are rated on a 4-point scale from strongly agree to disagree:

- *It helps me do what I want*—this captures whether the product is useful in helping you achieve your aims.
- *It is easy to use*—this rates user experience.
- *I can get help if I need it*—this rates the availability of support either from other people or online.
- *I am satisfied with this product*—this rates overall satisfaction with the product. This is intended to be a broader concept than the previous items.

Behaviour Change

Many innovations are intended to promote or require behaviour change. For behaviour to take place, each user must have the capability, opportunity and sufficiently strong motivation to do it. This is the COM-B model, which is essentially bottom-up, focusing on those whose behaviour is targeted, why and how people change their behaviour. It helps us understand how to introduce changes in behaviour and culture successfully at the level of individuals, communities and populations, or why the behaviour change that was expected did not occur [8].

Capability The person or people must have the physical strength, knowledge, skills, stamina etc. to perform the behaviour.

Opportunity The behaviour must be physically accessible, affordable, socially acceptable and people be given sufficient time to do it.

Motivation People must be more strongly motivated to do the behaviour at the relevant time than not to do it, or do something else. Motivation includes both unconscious habits (automatic) and conscious (reflective) thoughts and goals,

Behaviour change

Thinking about this behaviour

	Strongly agree	Agree	Neutral	Disagree
I have the skills and/or tools needed	😀	🙂	😐	☹️
Nothing stops me from doing it	😀	🙂	😐	☹️
I choose to do it	😀	🙂	😐	☹️
I do it without thinking	😀	🙂	😐	☹️

Fig. 16.5 Behaviour change measure

corresponding to fast automatic thinking (Kahneman's System 1) and slow reflective thinking (System 2) [15].

Both capability and opportunity impact motivation; these impact behaviour and, in turn, are impacted by behaviour change. To change behaviour, you must be clear about what behaviour you seek as well as the context in which it can be achieved. Then think about what must change, by and with whom, where, when and how often. For one type of behaviour change it may be best to remove a perceived barrier by enabling capability, while for another it may be better to deter behaviour by restricting the opportunity to do it.

The Behaviour Change measure contains one item on capability, one on opportunity and two about motivation (reflective and automatic) (Fig. 16.5).

Training

Education and training enable health and care staff to provide appropriate care and treatment, and patients to look after their own conditions whenever possible. An enormous amount of resource is devoted to education and training patients and staff in the health and care services. Training is invariably an important component in successful innovation spread.

There is an obvious need to evaluate all training and education activities in terms of their impact on students, such as whether they do the right things and do them well. Our focus here is on training, where the dominant approach for about 60 years has been the Kirkpatrick Model [8].

Kirkpatrick defines four levels or dimensions: *Reaction*, *Learning*, *Behaviour* and *Results*. Each level is important and has an impact on the next level.

Reaction—*It was relevant and I enjoyed it*—this is the level of participant satisfaction with the course. This is always important if participants are to engage fully in the course.

Learning—*I have learnt new things*—this is the extent to which participants improve knowledge, mindset or expertise as a result of attending the program. This often measured using formal tests and assessments, sometimes on a before and after basis. The learning objectives should be specifically defined.

Behaviour—*I shall use what I have learnt*—this is the extent to which change in behaviour takes place because of the training program. Behaviour change depends on capabilities, opportunity and motivation (the COM-B model, see above). It is sometimes suggested that change in Behaviour should not be evaluated until 3–6 months after training, but this is often not practicable.

Results—*The impact on my work should be good*—this is the outcome which occurs because the participants attend the program. The idea is to determine if the material has a positive impact of the participants' organisation, family etc. Impact on an organisation or business may include improved quality, safety and compliance, fewer accidents, reduced waste and staff turnover. From a payer's point of view, the main reason for funding training programs is usually to achieve these end results. However, training results are notoriously difficult to measure because what is measured is typically long term and impacted by many other influences.

Working with healthcare services who have introduced new ways of working, we recognised that training is a key aspect of the change management process for staff and an important aspect of treatment for patients. We saw a way to measure training outcomes based on Kirkpatrick's four levels, based on the design criteria, outlined earlier. This led to a measure that is much shorter and simpler than previous proposals, as shown in Fig. 16.6.

Training

Thinking about this course

	Strongly agree	Agree	Neutral	Disagree
It was relevant and I enjoyed it	😀	🙂	😐	☹️
I have learnt new things	😀	🙂	😐	☹️
I shall use what I have learnt	😀	🙂	😐	☹️
The impact on my work should be good	😀	🙂	😐	☹️

Fig. 16.6 Training

Digital Competence

Digital competence is competence to adopt, use and spread digital healthcare technologies effectively. This measure (Fig. 16.7) is mainly for health care staff, to help managers assess the readiness of their organisation to adopt new digital innovations. The first two items are related to enthusiasm to embrace new innovations, while the third and fourth items are about support and self-efficacy.

It is important to recognise that this measure is product-specific. Different products or applications may get different answers. For example, some people may be perfectly happy with what they already use but resist any calls for them to take on new products.

Product Confidence

It is important that people are confident to use innovative products. The Product Confidence measure asks about frequency of use, confidence and knowledge of the benefits and possible problems associated with its use (Fig. 16.8). This is complementary to the product satisfaction measure (above).

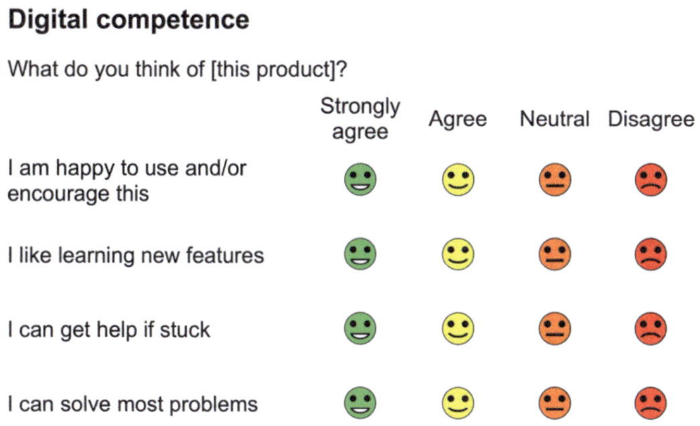

Digital competence

What do you think of [this product]?

	Strongly agree	Agree	Neutral	Disagree
I am happy to use and/or encourage this	😀	🙂	😐	☹️
I like learning new features	😀	🙂	😐	☹️
I can get help if stuck	😀	🙂	😐	☹️
I can solve most problems	😀	🙂	😐	☹️

Fig. 16.7 Digital competence measure

Product confidence

What do you feel about using this product?

	Strongly agree	Agree	Neutral	Disagree
I use it frequently	😀	🙂	😐	🙁
I feel confident using it	😀	🙂	😐	🙁
I know about the benefits	😀	🙂	😐	🙁
I know about the problems	😀	🙂	😐	🙁

Fig. 16.8 Product confidence measure

Case Study—Digital Readiness in General Practice

General practice surgeries in the UK rapidly adopted computers during the period between 1987 and 1994, but since then progress has been slow and variable. Reports of rapid change since the start of the COVID pandemic may be over-optimistic, due to issues in IT infrastructure, software usability, interoperability and information governance that have not been fully resolved.

The aim of this case study was to understand how different factors—technologies, patients, staff, practice culture and external factors impact digital readiness within general practice. A full report on this project is available [16].

A digital readiness survey tool was developed and used in a sample of 27 general practices (339 GPs, nurses and non-clinical staff) in north and mid Hampshire, England, between February and June 2020.

The study focused on five digital healthcare technologies. Two were staff facing—electronic patient records (EPR) and telehealth applications (text messaging and video consultations); three were patient-facing—patient online access, patient apps and wearables, and social media.

The survey results guided semi-structured qualitative interviews (n = 9) with some practice staff and digital technology company representatives. The survey mainly used variants of the digital competence measure (described above) plus relevant information about job, age and practice.

Key findings from the study were that younger staff and those in post for five or less years were more competent than older staff in most technologies. This applied to both clinical and non-clinical staff.

Large differences were found between the five technologies examined.

Technologies that directly benefited staff were well liked. These include EPRs that allow GPs to process prescriptions quickly, telehealth applications that help manage remote consultations, and patient access that allows patients to review their own test results and to book appointments.

However, patient apps and wearables, and self-help social media groups were regarded less favourably. There was a broad feeling that these technologies added risks and delivered few benefits. Younger staff were far more enthusiastic about these technologies than older staff.

Across all technologies, the lowest scores were for *Ability to solve problems if stuck*, which highlighted the need for more and better training and support.

Perhaps unexpectedly, this study found that practices with more deprived populations were more enthusiastic about digital technology than those in affluent areas. Practices with an older patient population, in the countryside and having a smaller practice size were usually less deprived and were less digitally enthusiastic. Their patients also tended to have poorer digital infrastructure, such as high speed internet.

This study illustrates the complexity of improving digital readiness in general practice. It is not simply a matter of having the best tools, although that helps. Innovation needs to be well-resourced and supported by digital implementation teams. More collaboration is also needed between technology companies, GPs, patients, and central and regional agencies.

Comparison of Measures

Table 16.1 compares the number of items, number of response options, word count, Flesch-Kincaid readability grade (FKG), and the range of scores possible for a group of people for each measure described in this chapter. This table shows similarities in the design of each measure.

Table 16.1 Comparison of measures showing: number of items, number of response options, recall period, word count, Flesch-Kincaid Grade (FKG) readability measure and possible range

Measure	Items	Options	Recall	Words	FKG	Range
Innovation readiness	4	4	Now	38	4.4	0 to 100
Digital confidence	4	4	Now	41	5.8	0 to 100
Innovation process	4	4	Now	42	3.6	0 to 100
User satisfaction	4	4	Now	38	1.3	0 to 100
Behaviour change	4	4	Now	32	3.9	0 to 100
Training	4	4	Now	35	1.8	0 to 100
Digital competence	4	4	Now	36	2.4	0 to 100
Product confidence	4	4	Now	31	4.6	0 to 100

Word count and FKG include the standard items, preamble, and options, but not the title or any copyright notices. Reading age is approximately FKG + 5. Range is the possible score range of values from floor to ceiling.

Conclusions

These short survey measures have been developed for use in evaluation of health and care innovations. They can be used individually or in combination or with other outcome and experience measures. These tools can also be used prospectively to identify people and organisations that are ready to adopt innovations and to help those less ready to become more prepared.

References

1. Kelley W. The evolution of laparoscopy and the revolution in surgery in the decade of the 1990s. JSLS. 2008;12:351–7.
2. Maguire D, Evans H, Honeyman M, Omojomolo D. Digital change in health and social care. London: The Kings Fund; 2018.
3. Braithwaite J, Churruca K, Long JC, et al. When complexity science meets implementation science: a theoretical and empirical analysis of systems change. BMC Med. 2018;16:63.
4. Greenhalgh T, Wherton J, Papoutsi C, et al. Beyond adoption: a new framework for theorising and evaluating non-adoption, abandonment and challenges to scale-up, spread and sustainability of health and care technologies. J Med Internet Res. 2017; 19(11):e367.
5. Rogers E. Diffusion of Innovations. 5th ed. New York NY: Free Press; 2003.
6. May C, Finch T. Implementing, embedding, and integrating practices: an outline of normalization process theory. Sociology. 2009;43(3):535–54.
7. Michie S, Atkins L, West R. The behaviour change wheel: a guide to designing interventions. London: Silverback Publishing; 2014.
8. Kirkpatrick DL, Kirkpatrick JD. Evaluating training programs: the four levels, 3rd ed. San Francisco CA: Berrett-Koehler;2006.
9. Heifetz R, Laurie D. The work of leadership. Harv Bus Rev. 2001:35–48.
10. Kontos E, Blake K, Chou W, Prestin A. Predictors of eHealth usage: insights on the digital divide from the health information national trends survey 2012. J Med Internet Res. 2014; 16(7):e172.
11. Tennant B, Stellefson M, Dodd V, et al. eHealth literacy and Web 2.0 health information seeking behaviors among baby boomers and older adults. J Med Internet Res. 2015; 17(3): e70.
12. Compeau D, Higgins C. Computer self-efficacy: development of a measure and initial test. MIS Q. 1995;19(2):189–211.
13. Finch T, Rapley T, Girling M, et al. Improving the normalization of complex interventions: measure development based on normalization process theory (NoMAD): study protocol. Implement Sci. 2013;8(1):43.
14. Stoyanov SR, Hides L, Kavanagh DJ, et al. Mobile app rating scale: a new tool for assessing the quality of health mobile apps. JMIR mHealth uHealth 2015; 3(1):e27.

15. Kahneman D. Thinking, fast and slow. New York: Farrar, Straus and Giroux; 2011.
16. Hammerton M, Sibley A, Benson T. Digital readiness within general practice. Southampton: Wessex AHSN;2021. https://wessexahsn.org.uk/img/news/Digital%20Readiness%20Study%20Report_full_report-1612545101.pdf. Accessed 23 Oct 2021.

Staff-Reported Measures 17

Background

Staff-reported and patient-reported measures cover the same domains, although there are important differences between them. It helps to consider these roles separately. Staff see many patients and the data collection process is simpler. Many staff-reported measures were adapted from patient-reported measures. Patients are subjects of care while staff provide care (e.g. clinicians, admin staff and volunteers) within an organisational structure.

Staff are good survey subjects for several reasons. It is often easier to ask staff to complete surveys and they have a better response rate than for patients, if only because staff tend to do what their line manager asks them to do. Staff understand how the system works in practice, rather than how it is intended to work. However, they may not wish to speak truth unto power, which is a reason for making staff responses anonymous.

Most staff joined the health and care services because they wanted to help people. They also want to help make it work better. Staff feel frustrated when policies and processes prevents quality improvement and like to have their voice heard.

This chapter contains some new material in addition to that previously published. [1] Patient-reported measures have been summarised in Chap. 9.

Table 17.1 provides a summary of the staff-reported measures listed below. It shows the measures and their items in three columns: the name, the text shown to respondents, the response option sets and relevant chapters.

The following option sets are used:

- None—Extreme (None, A little, Quite a lot, Extreme)
- Strongly agree—Disagree (Strongly agree, Agree, Neutral, Disagree)
- Excellent—Poor (Excellent, Good, Fair, Poor).

Quality of Life

Staff health and wellbeing is always important and has become even more so since the start of the pandemic. Burnout—a syndrome of exhaustion, depersonalization and reduced professional efficacy—is always a risk for health and care staff, and COVID has substantially increased this risk [2].

These quality of life measures are about the respondent themselves.

Health Status
The health status measure for staff (*howRu*) is the same as that used for patients [3] (See also Chap. 11).

Work Wellbeing
The Work Wellbeing Score is focused on the respondent's view of their job and is based closely on the Personal Wellbeing Score (PWS) [4] (See also Chap. 12).

Person-Specific Outcome
The individualised person specific outcome measure gives staff an opportunity to list two issues that they would like to be addressed [5] (See also Chap. 14).

Individual Care

Job Confidence
The Job Confidence Score focuses on how confident people feel in their work role. It provides staff with an opportunity to indicate their confidence in doing their job and the level of support they are getting. Job confidence (JCS) was adapted from the health confidence score [6] (See also Chap. 13).

Assessed Need
Staff or carer assessment of patients with dementia or frailty being cared for at home or in residential care homes [7].

Care Provided

Experience Care provided covers both individual services and the way that services work together. Patients and staff have views about the quality of care provided.

Service Provided
Service experience (staff) asks how staff perceive the service their team provides. Adapted from the *howRwe* experience measure [4] (See also Chap. 10).

Service Integration
Service integration (staff) asks how staff perceive collaboration with other services. Staff perceptions often differ from those of patients. (See also Chap. 10).

Patient Confidence
Patient confidence asks how staff perceive patients' health confidence as a population. If staff report on individuals, they should use HCS as a proxy [6] (See also Chap. 13).

Provider Culture

Provider culture measures aspects of each health and care organisation's policies and practice. Culture is all important. As Peter Drucker once said: "Culture eats policy for breakfast".

Staff, who work in an organization, invariably have better direct knowledge and experience of the culture than can patients, who are only occasional visitors.

PREMs can assess many aspects of culture. We have focused on staff relationships, shared decision-making, patient safety, staff safety and privacy.

Traditionally, health and care services have had clear demarcations between the role played by different professions and specialties, which have been jealously guarded by trade unions and professional societies.

Staff Relationships
Staff relationships impact on how well different groups of people work together for a common good, as explored by Gittell's work on relational coordination [8].

Shared Decisions
Shared decisions (staff) address staff perceptions of shared decision-making in general, as opposed to that for individual patients [9] (See also Chap. 13).

Patient Safety
Patient safety focuses on clinical aspects of safety including adverse events and cultural attitudes towards safety and learning from incidents [10].

Staff Safety
Staff safety. Staff need to feel safe from being attacked by patients or bullied by managers within the organisation and outside [11].

Privacy
Privacy covers patients and staff perceptions of information governance including data protection, data sharing, subject access and satisfaction [12].

Innovation

Innovation focuses on the impact of specific innovations, such as digital health applications and new ways of working [13]. Staff are invariably involved and patients less frequently (See also Chap. 16).

Innovation Readiness
Innovation readiness (staff) covers where people and organisations fall on the innovativeness spectrum [14].

Innovation Process
Innovation process is based on May's Normalisation Process Theory (NPT) in terms of how well innovations are implemented [15].

User Satisfaction
User satisfaction focuses on people's perception of how much an innovation is useful and easy to use, availability of help and overall satisfaction [16].

Behaviour Change
Behaviour change covers capability, opportunity and motivation (conscious and unconscious) to change behaviour based on Michie's COM-B model [17].

Training
The Training measure is based on Kirkpatrick, who defines four levels or dimensions: Reaction, Learning, Behaviour and Results [18].

Digital Competence
Staff digital confidence assesses people's confidence in using digital apps and similar devices at work [13].

Product Confidence
Product confidence covers staff understanding of and confidence to use a specific innovation, application or product [13].

Table 17.1 Staff-Reported Measures

Name	Text used in survey	Options
Quality of life		
Health status	How are you today? (past 24 h)	None–extreme
Pain/discomfort	Pain or discomfort	Chapter 11
Distress	Feeling low or worried	
Disability	Limited in what you can do	
Dependence	Require help from others	
Work wellbeing	How content are you in your job?	Strongly agree–disagree

(continued)

Table 17.1 (continued)

Name	Text used in survey	Options
Job satisfaction	I am satisfied with my job	Chapter 12
Worthwhile job	I am valued for what I do	
Happy at work	I was happy yesterday* at work	
Not anxious at work	I was NOT anxious yesterday* at work	
Person specific outcome	List one or two issues you would like help with	None–extreme
Issue 1	Issue 1 [write in]	Chapter 14
Issue 2	Issue 2 [write in]	
Individual care		
Job confidence	How confident do you feel in your job?	Strongly agree–disagree
Knowledge	I know enough about my job	Chapter 13
Self-management	I can manage my work	
Access to help	I can get help if I need it	
Shared decisions	I am involved in decisions that affect me	
Assessed need	How are they doing?	None–extreme**
Physical needs	Physical care needs	
Distress	Pain and/or distress	
Unpredictable	Unpredictable needs	
Challenging	Behaviour problems	
Care provided		
Service provided	What do you think about the service we provide?	Excellent–poor
We are kind	Treat people kindly	Chapter 10
We listen/explain	Listen and explain	
We are prompt	See people promptly	
Well organised	Well organised	
Service integration	How do you work with other services?	Strongly agree–disagree
Services talk together	Services talk to each other	Chapter 10
Service knowledge	We know what other services do	
Care planning	We consider other services when planning care	
Part of team	We feel part of the overall care team	
Patient confidence	How confident are patients in caring for their health?	Strongly agree–disagree
Patient knowledge	They know enough about their health	Chapter 13
Self-management	They can look after their health	
Patient access	They can get the help they need	

(continued)

Table 17.1 (continued)

Name	Text used in survey	Options
Shared decisions	They are involved in decisions about themselves	
Provider culture		
Staff relationships	*Thinking about colleagues in other services*	Strongly agree–disagree
We know each other	We know each other	
Rely on each other	We rely on each other	
Share information	We share information	
Help each other	We help each other	
Shared decisions	*Thinking about your patients' choices*	Strongly agree–disagree
Patients know benefits	They know the possible benefits	Chapter 13
Patients know risks	They know the possible downside	
Patients know choices	They know that they have choices	
Fully involved	They are fully involved	
Patient safety	*Thinking about patient safety*	Strongly agree–disagree
Adverse events	Adverse events are rare	
Systems are safe	Our systems are safe	
Open about errors	We are open if things go wrong	
Learn from mistakes	We learn from our mistakes	
Staff safety	*Thinking about your own safety*	Strongly agree–disagree
Safe at work	I feel safe at work	
Respected at work	I feel respected at work	
Safe outside	I feel safe outside work	
Respected outside	I feel respected outside work	
Privacy	*Thinking about how we use patient data*	Strongly agree–disagree
Data is safe	Patient data is kept safe and secure	
Shared as needed	Patient data is only shared as needed	
Patients check data	Patients can see and check their data	
Happy about data use	I am happy about how patient data is used	
Innovation		Chapter 16
Innovation readiness	*New ideas in your field of work*	Strongly agree–disagree
New ideas needed	New ideas are needed in my field	Chapter 16
Keep up to date	I keep up with new ideas	

(continued)

Table 17.1 (continued)

Name	Text used in survey	Options
We back new ideas	My organisation supports new ideas	
We make ideas work	My organisation makes new ideas work	
Innovation Process	*Thinking about [this project]*	Strongly agree–disagree
Vision is followed	The original vision is being followed	Chapter 16
Plan to make it work	We all thought about how to make it work	
We work together	We all act to make it work	
Reflection	We all think about how to keep it going	
User satisfaction	*What do you think of [this product]?*	Strongly agree–disagree
Helps me	It helps me do what I want	Chapter 16
Easy to use	It is easy to use	
Can get help	I can get help if I need it	
Product satisfaction	I am satisfied with this product	
Behaviour change	*Thinking about [this behaviour]*	Strongly agree–disagree
Capability	I am able to do it (skills and tools)	Chapter 16
Opportunity	Nothing prevents me from doing it	
Conscious motive	I choose to do it	
Automatic motive	I do it without thinking	
Training	*Thinking about this course*	Strongly agree–disagree
Reaction	It was relevant and I enjoyed it	Chapter 16
Learning	I have learnt new things	
Behaviour	I shall use what I have learnt	
Results	The impact on my work should be good	
Digital competence	*What do you think of [this product]*	Strongly agree–disagree
IT confidence	I am happy to use and/or encourage this	Chapter 16
Learning apps	I enjoy learning new features	
Can get help	I can get help if I stuck	
Solve IT problems	I can solve most problems	
Product confidence	*How do you feel about using [this product]?*	Strongly agree–disagree
Frequent user	I use it frequently	Chapter 16
Confident user	I feel confident using it	
Know benefits	I know about the benefits	
Know problems	I know about the problems	

* Work wellbeing: previous working day
** Assessed need: quite a lot needs 1 person most of the time; extreme needs 2 people

References

1. Benson T. Measure what we want: a taxonomy of short generic person-reported outcome and experience measures (PROMs and PREMs). BMJ Open Qual. 2020; 9:e000789.
2. Denning M, Goh ET, Tan B, et al. Determinants of burnout and other aspects of psychological well-being in healthcare workers during the Covid-19 pandemic: a multinational cross-sectional study. PLoS ONE 2021; 16(4):e0238666.
3. Benson T, Whatling J, Arikan S, McDonald D, Ingram D. Evaluation of a new short generic measure of HRQoL: howRu. Inform Prim Care. 2010; 18:89–101.
4. Benson T, Potts HWW. A short generic patient experience questionnaire: howRwe development and validation. BMC Health Serv Res. 2014; 14:499.
5. Benson T. Person-specific outcome measure (PSO) for use in primary and community care. BMJ Open Qual. 2021; 10:e001379.
6. Benson T, Potts HWW, Bark P, et al. Development and initial testing of a Health Confidence Score (HCS). BMJ Open Qual. 2019; 8:e000411.
7. Algase DL, Beck C, Kolanowski A, et al. Need-driven dementia-compromised behavior: an alternative view of disruptive behavior. Am J Alzheimers Dis. 1996; 11(6):10–9.
8. Gittell JH. Transforming relationships for high performance: the power of relational coordination. San Francisco CA: Stanford Business Books; 2016.
9. Barry MJ, Edgman-Levitan S. Shared decision making—the pinnacle of patient-centered care. N Engl J Med. 2012; 366(9):780–1.
10. Gandhi TK, Kaplan GS, Leape L, et al. Transforming concepts in patient safety: a progress report. BMJ Qual. Saf. 2018; 27:1019–26.
11. Privitera M, Weisman R, Cerulli C, et al. Violence toward mental health staff and safety in the work environment. Occup Med. 2005; 55(6):480–6.
12. van Staa T-P, Goldacre B, Buchan I, et al. Big health data: the need to earn public trust. BMJ 2016; 354:i3636.
13. Benson T. Digital innovation evaluation: user perceptions of innovation readiness, digital confidence, innovation adoption, user experience and behaviour change. BMJ Health Care Inform. 2019; 26:000018.
14. Rogers EM. Diffusion of innovations, 5th ed. Mumbai: The Free Press; 2003.
15. May CR, Mair F, Finch T, et al. Development of a theory of implementation and integration: normalization process theory. Implement Sci. 2009;4(1):29.
16. Stoyanov S, Hides L, Kavanagh D, et al. Mobile app rating scale: a new tool for assessing the quality of health mobile apps. JMIR Mhealth Uhealth 2015; 3(1):e27.
17. Michie S, Van Stralen MM, West R. The behaviour change wheel: a new method for characterising and designing behaviour change interventions. Implement Sci. 2011;6(1):42.
18. Kirkpatrick DL, Kirkpatrick JD. Evaluating training programs: the four levels, 3rd ed. San Francisco CA: Berrett-Koehler; 2006.

Proxies, Caregivers and Care Home Residents

Proxies

In some cases, people cannot complete PROMs and PREMs reliably. For example, children may be too young to complete PROMs reliably; people living with stroke, head injury or dementia may have physical or mental impairments that prevent them from competing surveys at all. When this happens it is better to collect data via a proxy than to have nothing.

Proxys can be quite reliable at assessing objective physical capabilities—what people can and cannot do for themselves. However, people who have adapted to living with disability for many years tend compare with their normal disabled selves, not with people without any disability. People in a specific environment, such as a ward or care home, tend to compare themselves with others in the same place or of the same age, not the staff. Patients frequently rate their own quality of life, in terms of function, as substantially higher than do proxies [1, 2].

People are much less good at assessing how other people are feeling. Ideally proxies should be relatives, partners, or friends, who know the patient well, rather than someone who has had little direct contact with the patient. People, who are closer to the patient, are usually better at recognising how someone is feeling, but even then people can be good at disguising their real feelings.

Staff in the role of proxy can be trained to rate people, but noise and bias are always risks (see Chap. 5). People acting as proxies should always try to agree their rating with the subject of the rating.

Caregivers

Unpaid caregivers, also known as carers, provide a vital role in helping people live in their own homes. They differ from paid care workers who care for people as part of their paid employment, such as care assistants, nurses and support workers. They provide a range of support including personal care, emotional support, help with practical task such as shopping and reminding or giving medication. Around 10% of the population provide unpaid care.

Case Study

This project set out to understand the perceptions of caregivers and those they care for in terms of wellbeing, health status and health confidence, in a GP practice near Windsor, England. It is unusual in comparing caregivers and cared for using very similar instruments. A short report on this study has been published previously [3].

Questions cover wellbeing, health status and confidence, using versions of the Personal Wellbeing Score (a short version of ONS4) [4], *howRu* (health status measure) [5], and Health Confidence Score [6]. These are described in Chaps. 11, 12 and 13. The questions were the same for both groups, with one exception – caregivers were asked *I know enough about caring* and those being cared were asked about *I know enough about my health*. The questions for caregivers are shown in Fig. 18.1.

Each question had four response options. If the person being cared for could not complete the survey, a proxy was allowed. Mean scores for each item, and mean

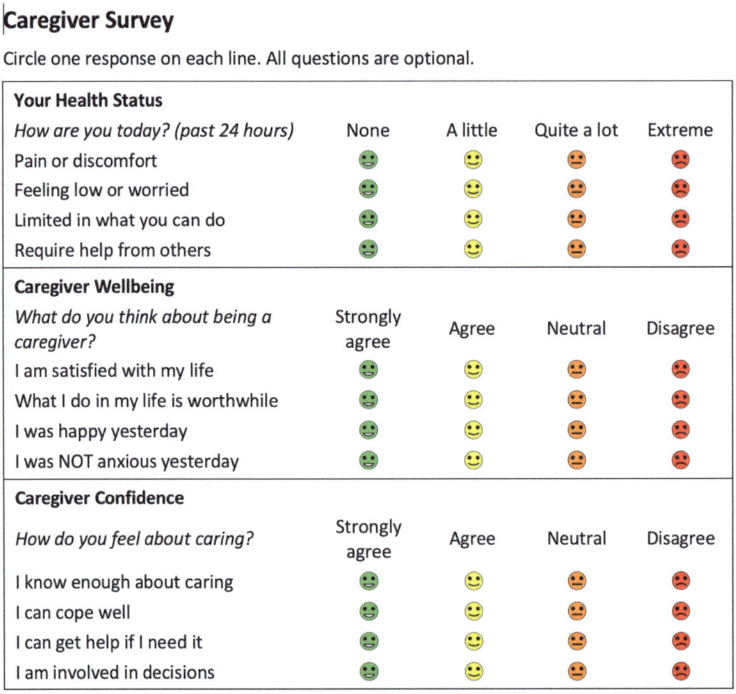

Fig. 18.1 Caregiver questionnaire

summary scores based on the average of items in a measure, are shown using a scale from 0 (all at floor) to 100 (all at ceiling).

Both caregivers and those they cared for had a similar gender split (60% female, 40% male); 8% of those being cared for were under 20; 53% were over 80; 57% of caregivers were over 70.

Table 18.1 shows the number of responses and mean scores for each measure's summary scores and item scores reported by caregivers and those they care for. The difference column shows the mean caregiver score minus the mean cared for score. Two stars indicates that the difference has less than 1% probability of occurring by chance; one star indicates that there is between 5 and 1% probability of occurring by chance.

When looking at these results it is important to consider both the magnitude of the scores and the differences between the scores for caregivers and those they care for. As a guide, scores over 80 are good, 60–79 are moderate, 40–59 are low and below 40 are very low.

Both groups are equally unhappy and anxious and perceive a need to know more. This indicates that these areas need more attention.

Caregivers have higher scores than those they care for disability (+27), dependence (+25), worthwhileness (+21), ability to cope (+16) although scores for both groups are low, and involvement in decisions (+14). The only item where caregivers scored lower than those they care for was for getting help when needed, although the difference was not significant and neither score was good.

Table 18.1 Number of responses and mean scores for measures and items reported by caregivers and those they care for

Measure	Caregiver		Cared for		Difference
	n	Score	n	Score	
Health status summary	93	72	88	58	14**
Pain or discomfort	96	73	91	68	6*
Feeling low or worried	95	69	88	67	2
Limited in what you can do	95	73	90	45	27**
Require help from others	93	74	90	49	25**
Wellbeing summary	94	57	88	50	8*
I am satisfied with my life	96	52	91	44	8*
What I do in my life is worthwhile	95	71	89	50	21**
I was happy yesterday	95	57	90	56	1
I was NOT anxious yesterday	94	50	89	50	0
Health confidence summary	93	62	90	55	8
I know enough about caring/my health	94	55	90	50	5
I can cope well	94	60	90	43	16**
I can get help if I need it	96	60	90	64	−3
I am involved in decisions	93	75	90	61	14**

This study has limitations. Sample size was small and it was done in only one GP practice.

These surveys were straight-forward to use and helped identify areas where caregiver support can be improved. Overall, one is left with the feeling that the main difference between caregivers and those they care for is that caregivers are less functionally disabled than those they care for but are equally unhappy. This is in alignment with other research [7].

Care Home Residents

Care home residents are amongst the most vulnerable people. A large proportion have dementia, frailty or learning disabilities, which mean that they cannot live on their own without support. The health status of care home residents is a key parameter for all concerned in care homes. A simple method to track health status routinely at both the individual and collectively at care home level is necessary to understand and optimize care and support decision-making.

In 2012, Bupa Care Services undertook a census of 24,506 residents in 395 care homes which they managed in UK, Australia and New Zealand and collected staff-reported health status, using the *howRu* measure [8]. This demonstrated the practicality of using this type of measure at scale in different countries. There were significant differences between staff ratings and those made by residents themselves. At more severe states, residents scored worse than staff for pain and distress, but staff scored worse than residents for disability and dependence [9].

A different study in care homes looked at staff reports of their work well-being, job confidence and perception of the care provided. This found that care homes that scored highly on these measures were also rated highly by independent inspectors [10].

References

1. Jones J, McPherson C, Zimmermann C, et al. Assessing agreement between terminally ill cancer patients' reports of their quality of life and family caregiver and palliative care physician proxy ratings. J Pain Symptom Manag. 2011; 42(3):354–65.
2. Williams L, Tamilyn Bakas T, Brizendine E, et al. How valid are family proxy assessments of stroke patients' health-related quality of life? Stroke. 2006; 37(8):2081–5.
3. Benson T, Walker C. Wellbeing, health status and confidence of carers and those cared for in a GP practice. Qual Life Res. 2018; 27(Suppl 1):S133.
4. Benson T, Sladen J, Liles A, Potts H. Personal Wellbeing Score (PWS)—a short version of ONS4, testing and validation in social prescribing. BMJ Open Qual. 2019; 8:e000394.
5. Benson T, Whatling J, Arikan S, Sizmur S, McDonald D, Ingram D. Evaluation of a new short generic measure of HRQoL: howRu. Inform Prim Care. 2010; 18:89–101.
6. Benson T, Potts HWW, Bark P, Bowman C. Development and initial testing of a health confidence score (HCS). BMJ Open Qual. 2019; 8:e000411.
7. Unpaid Care. London: Parliamentary Office of Science and Technology POSTnote 582; 2018.

8. Benson T, Bowman C. Health status of care home residents: practicality and construct validity of data collection by staff at scale. BMJ Open Qual. 2019; 8:e000704.
9. Benson T, Bowman C. Comparison of staff and resident health status ratings in care homes. BMJ Open Qual. 2020; 9:e000801.
10. Benson T, Sladen J, Done J, Bowman C. Monitoring work well-being, job confidence and care provided by care home staff using a self-report survey. BMJ Open Qual. 2019; 8: e000621.

Appendix

This Appendix lists LOINC and SNOMED CT codes, which have been developed for some of the PROMs and PREMs described in this book. These codes are designed to be used in two related use cases. First, to enable interoperability, where information needs to be moved from one computer system to another in a way that both ends understand. Secondly, where the requirement is to store data in a vendor-independent way, such as on a patient portal, where it can be read by different systems.

The lists shown here are summaries of the more extensive documentation available on the LOINC and SNOMED web sites. In some places the local preference is to use LOINC for these use cases, in other places the preference is to use SNOMED CT.

LOINC Codes

Table A1 contains a list of LOINC codes contained in the loinc.csv and LoincAnswerlistLink.csv files (version 2.72 February 2022). For full details see the latest LOINC release files at https://loinc.org. Other codes will be added in later releases.

LOINC Answers

Many measures use the same option sets, which are documented in LOINC using Answer lists, Answer strings and Answer codes (Table A2). The Value for individual ratings is also shown.

SNOMED CT Codes

The SNOMED CT Codes shown in Table A3 are extension concept codes. Those containing the string "100000010" are UK codes. Those containing the string "100028610" are managed by R-Outcomes.

© The Editor(s) (if applicable) and The Author(s), under exclusive license to Springer Nature Switzerland AG 2022
T. Benson, *Patient-Reported Outcomes and Experience*,
https://doi.org/10.1007/978-3-030-97071-0

Table A1 LOINC codes showing name LOINC code Item name property and answer list. The question preamble is shown in parentheses)

Name	LOINC code	Item (Question preamble)	Prop	Answer list
Health status (howRu)	55744–7	howRu panel (How are you today? (past 24 h))	Panel	
howRu summary score	55749–6	howRu score	Score	
Pain or discomfort	55745–4	How are you today: pain or discomfort	Find	LL755-0
Feeling low or worried	55746–2	How are you today: feeling low or worried	Find	LL755-0
Limited in what you can do	55747–0	How are you today: limited in what I can do	Find	LL755-0
Require help from others	55748–8	Require help from others	Find	LL755-0
Personal well-being score (PWS)	96929–5	Personal well-being panel (How are you feeling in general)	Panel	
PWS summary score	96930–3	Personal well-being score	Score	
I am satisfied with my life	96931–1	I am satisfied with my life	Find	LL5780-3
What I do in my life is worthwhile	96932–9	What I do in my life is worthwhile	Find	LL5780-3
I was happy yesterday	96933–7	I was happy yesterday	Find	LL5780-3
I was NOT anxious yesterday	96934–5	I was not anxious yesterday	Find	LL5780-3
Sleep	97890–8	Sleep panel (Thinking about your recent sleep pattern)	Panel	
Sleep score	97891–6	Sleep score	Score	
Sleep at same time	97892–4	Go to sleep at the same time	Find	LL5780-3
Wake at same time	97893–2	Wake up at the same time	Find	LL5780-3
Wake refreshed	97894–0	Wake up feeling refreshed	Find	LL5780-3
Sleep well	97895–7	Sleep well	Find	LL5780-3
Fatigue	97902–1	Fatigue panel (Thinking about getting tired)	Panel	
Fatigue score	97903–9	Fatigue total score	Score	
Energy level	97904–7	Usually have enough energy	Find	LL5780-3
Tire quickly	97905–4	Do not tire too quickly	Find	LL5780-3
Able to concentrate	97906–2	Usually concentrate well	Find	LL5780-3

(continued)

Table A1 (continued)

Name	LOINC code	Item (Question preamble)	Prop	Answer list
Stamina	97907-0	Can keep going if needed	Find	LL5780-3
Health confidence	96945-1	Health confidence panel (How do you feel about caring for your health)	Panel	
HCS	96946-9	Health confidence score	Score	
Knowledge	96950-1	I know enough about my health	Find	LL5780-3
Self-management	96947-7	I can look after my health	Find	LL5780-3
Access to help	96948-5	I can get the right help if I need it	Find	LL5780-3
Shared decisions	96949-3	I am involved in decisions about me	Find	LL5780-3
Self-care	97896-5	Self-care panel (How well do you look after yourself?)	Panel	
Self-care score	97897-3	Self-care total score	Score	
Diet management	97898-1	Manage diet well	Find	LL5780-3
Exercise management	97899-9	Manage physical activity well	Find	LL5780-3
Weight management	97900-5	Manage weight well	Find	LL5780-3
Meds management	97901-3	Manage medication well	Find	LL5780-3
Shared decisions	99417-8	Shared decision-making panel (Thinking about (your plan))	Panel	
SDM score	99418-6	Shared decision-making total score	Score	
Know benefits	99419-4	Know possible benefits of treatment plan	Find	LL5780-3
Know downside	99420-2	Know possible downside of treatment plan	Find	LL5780-3
Know choices	99421-0	Know available choices for treatment plan	Find	LL5780-3
Fully involved	99422-8	Feel fully involved in treatment plan	Find	LL5780-3
Behaviour change	99556-3	Behavior change panel (Thinking about (this behaviour))	Panel	
Behaviour change score	99557-1	Behavior change total score	Score	
Capability	99558-9	Skills and tools to change behavior	Find	LL5780-3
Opportunity	99559-7	Nothing prevents behavior change	Find	LL5780-3
Conscious motive	99560-5	Choose to change behavior	Find	LL5780-3
Automatic motive	99561-3	Change behavior without thinking	Find	LL5780-3
Adherence	99562-1	Adherence panel (Do you follow treatment instructions?)	Panel	

(continued)

Table A1 (continued)

Name	LOINC code	Item (Question preamble)	Prop	Answer list
Adherence score	99563–9	Adherence total score	Score	
Remember	99564–7	Remember to follow treatment instructions	Find	LL5780-3
Go on if I feel bad	99565–4	Follow treatment instructions if feel bad	Find	LL5780-3
Go on if I feel better	99566–2	Follow treatment instructions if feel better	Find	LL5780-3
Treatment satisfaction		Satisfaction with treatment	Find	LL5780-3
Acceptance of loss	99567–0	Acceptance of loss panel (Have you learnt to live with what's happened?)	Panel	
Acceptance of loss score	99568–8	Acceptance of loss total score	Score	
New capability	99569–6	Know capabilities following loss	Find	LL5780-3
Recognize loss	99570–4	Recognize life changes following loss	Find	LL5780-3
Change activity	99571–2	Activities done differently following loss	Find	LL5780-3
Move on	99572–0	Moved on following loss	Find	LL5780-3
Person specific measure	96936–0	Person-specific outcome panel (List one or two issues you would like help with)	Panel	
Issue (for each issue)	96937–8	Issue you would like help with	Find	
Score (for each issue)	96938–6	How much concern does the issue you would like help with cause	Find	LL5793-6
SDoH	96951–9	Social determinants of health panel (Thinking about how you live)	Panel	
SDoH score	96952–7	Social determinants of health score	Score	
Education	96953–5	I have had a good education	Find	LL1626-2
Autonomy	96954–3	I am valued for what I do	Find	LL1626-2
Housing	96955–0	I am happy about where I live	Find	LL1626-2
Enough money	96956–8	I have enough money to cope	Find	LL1626-2
Social contact	96939–4	Social contact panel (Thinking about your friends and family)	Panel	
Social contact score	96940–2	Social contact score	Score	
People to talk to	96941–0	I have people to talk to	Find	LL5780-3
People to confide in	96942–8	I have someone I can confide in	Find	LL5780-3
People to help	96943–6	I have people who will help me	Find	LL5780-3
	96944–4	I do things with others	Find	LL5780-3

(continued)

Appendix

Table A1 (continued)

Name	LOINC code	Item (Question preamble)	Prop	Answer list
Do things with others				
Patient experience	96783–6	howRwe panel (How are we doing? (our recent care))	Panel	
howRwe score	96784–4	howRwe score	Score	
Kindness	96785–1	Treat you kindly	Find	LL5784-5
Listen/explain	96786–9	Listen and explain	Find	LL5784-5
Prompt	96787–7	See you promptly	Find	LL5784-5
Organised	96788–5	Well organised	Find	LL5784-5
Service integration	96771–1	Service integration panel (How well do services work together)	Panel	
Integration score	96772–9	Service integration total score	Score	
Services talk together	96773–7	Services talk to each other	Find	LL5780-3
Service knowledge	96774–5	Staff know what other services do	Find	LL5780-3
Repeat story	96775–2	I don't have to repeat my story	Find	LL5780-3
Services work together	96776–0	Different services work well together	Find	LL5780-3

Table A2 LOINC Answer Lists

Answer list	Answer string	Answer code	Value
LL755-0	None	LA137-2	3
	A little	LA13940-4	2
	Quite a lot	LA11911-7	1
	Extreme	LA11912-5	0
LL5780-3	Strongly agree	LA15237-3	3
	Agree	LA15774-5	2
	Neutral	LA14786-0	1
	Disagree	LA15773-7	0
LL5784-5	Excellent	LA9206-9	3
	Good	LA8967-7	2
	Fair	LA8968-5	1
	Poor	LA8969-3	0
LL1626-2	Strongly agree	LA15237-3	3
	Agree	LA15774-5	2
	Disagree	LA15773-7	1
	Strongly disagree	LA15236-5	0

Table A3 SNOMED CT UK and R-Outcomes extension concept codes

Name	SCT ConceptId	Preferred synonym	Hierarchy
Health status (howRu)	515381000000104	howRu rating scale (How are you today? (past 24 h))	Assessment scale
howRu summary score	515461000000100	howRu rating score	Observable entity
Pain or discomfort	1038251000000103	Pain or discomfort	Observable entity
Feeling low or worried	1038231000000105	Feeling low or worried	Observable entity
Limited in what you can do	1038241000000101	Limited in what I can do	Observable entity
Require help from others	1038221000000108	Require help from others	Observable entity
Personal well-being score (PWS)	1053471000000102	Personal well-being panel (How are you feeling in general)	Assessment scale
PWS summary score	1053461000000109	Personal well-being score	Observable entity
I am satisfied with my life	1053421000000101	I am satisfied with my life	Observable entity
What I do in my life is worthwhile	1053431000000104	What I do in my life is worthwhile	Observable entity
I was happy yesterday	1053441000000108	I was happy yesterday	Observable entity
I was not anxious yesterday	1053451000000106	I was NOT anxious yesterday	Observable entity
Sleep	1011000286109	Sleep panel (Thinking about your recent sleep pattern)	Assessment scale
Sleep score	1021000286101	Sleep score	Observable entity
Sleep at same time	1031000286104	I go to sleep at the same time	Observable entity
Wake at same time	1041000286105	I wake up at the same time	Observable entity
Wake refreshed	1051000286108	I wake up feeling refreshed	Observable entity
Sleep well	1061000286106	I sleep well	Observable entity
Fatigue	1071000286102	Fatigue panel (Thinking about getting tired)	Assessment scale
Fatigue score	1081000286100	Fatigue total score	Observable entity
Energy level	1091000286103	I usually have enough energy	Observable entity

(continued)

Table A3 (continued)

Name	SCT ConceptId	Preferred synonym	Hierarchy
Tire quickly	1101000286108	I do not tire too quickly	Observable entity
Able to concentrate	1111000286105	I can usually concentrate well	Observable entity
Stamina	1121000286102	I can keep going if I need to	Observable entity
Health confidence	1001000286107	Health confidence panel (How do you feel about caring for your health?)	Assessment scale
HCS	1038201000000104	Health confidence score	Observable entity
Knowledge	1038141000000106	I know enough about my health	Observable entity
Self-management	1038121000000104	I can look after my health	Observable entity
Access to help	1038161000000107	I can get the right help if I need it	Observable entity
Shared decisions	1038181000000103	I am involved in decisions about me	Observable entity
Self–care	1131000286100	Self-care panel (How well do you look after yourself?)	Assessment scale
Self-care score	1141000286106	Self-care total score	Observable entity
Diet management	1151000286109	I can manage my diet	Observable entity
Exercise management	1161000286107	I can manage my physical activity	Observable entity
Weight management	1171000286103	I can manage my weight	Observable entity
Meds management	1181000286101	I can manage my medication	Observable entity
Shared decisions	1191000286104	Shared decision-making panel (Thinking about (your plan))	Assessment scale
SDM score	1201000286102	Shared decision-making total score	Observable entity
Know benefits	1211000286100	I know the possible benefits	Observable entity
Know downside	1221000286108	I know the possible downside	Observable entity
Know choices	1231000286105	I know that I have choices	Observable entity
Fully involved	1241000286104	I feel fully involved	Observable entity

(continued)

Table A3 (continued)

Name	SCT ConceptId	Preferred synonym	Hierarchy
Behaviour change	1251000286101	Behavior change panel (Thinking about (this behaviour))	Assessment scale
Behaviour change score	1261000286103	Behavior change score	Observable entity
Capability	1271000286107	I have the skills and tools to do it	Observable entity
Opportunity	1281000286109	Nothing prevents me from doing it	Observable entity
Conscious motive	1291000286106	I choose to do it	Observable entity
Automatic motive	1301000286105	I do it without thinking	Observable entity
Adherence	1311000286107	Adherence panel (Do you follow treatment instructions?)	Assessment scale
Adherence score	1321000286104	Adherence score	Observable entity
Remember	1331000286102	I remember to do it	Observable entity
Go on if I feel bad	1341000286108	I don't stop if I feel bad	Observable entity
Go on if I feel better	1351000286106	I don't stop if I feel better	Observable entity
Treatment satisfaction	1361000286109	I am happy with my treatment	Observable entity
Acceptance of loss	1371000286100	Acceptance of loss panel (Have you learnt to live with what's happened?)	Assessment scale
Acceptance of loss score	1381000286103	Acceptance of loss total score	Observable entity
New capability	1391000286101	I know what I can and cannot do	Observable entity
Recognise loss	1401000286103	I see how my life has changed	Observable entity
Change activity	1411000286101	I do things differently now	Observable entity
Move on	1421000286109	I have moved on	Observable entity
Person specific measure	1431000286106	Person-specific outcome panel (List one or two issues you would like help with)	Assessment scale
Issue (for each issue)	1441000286100	Issue you would like help with	Observable entity

(continued)

Table A3 (continued)

Name	SCT ConceptId	Preferred synonym	Hierarchy
Score (for each issue)	1451000286102	How much concern does the issue you would like help with cause	Observable entity
SDoH	1471000286108	Social determinants of health panel (Thinking about how you live)	Assessment scale
SDoH score	1481000286105	Social determinants of health score	Observable entity
Education	1491000286107	I have had a good education	Observable entity
Autonomy	1501000286104	I am in control of what I do	Observable entity
Housing	1511000286102	I am happy about where I live	Observable entity
Enough money	1521000286105	I have enough money to cope	Observable entity
Social contact	1531000286107	Social contact panel (Thinking about your friends and family)	Assessment scale
Social contact score	1541000286101	Social contact score	Observable entity
People to talk to	1551000286103	I have people to talk to	Observable entity
People to confide in	1561000286100	I have someone I can confide in	Observable entity
People to help	1571000286109	I have people who will help me	Observable entity
Do things with others	1581000286106	I do things with others	Observable entity
Neighbour relationships	1591000286108	Neighbour relationships panel (Thinking about your neighbours)	Assessment scale
Neighbour relationships score	1601000286100	Neighbour relationships score	Observable entity
Know each other	1611000286103	We know each other	Observable entity
Trust each other	1621000286106	We trust each other	Observable entity
Share information	1631000286108	We share information	Observable entity
Help each other	1641000286102	We help each other	Observable entity

(continued)

Table A3 (continued)

Name	SCT ConceptId	Preferred synonym	Hierarchy
Personal safety	1651000286104	Personal safety panel (Thinking about your own safety)	Assessment scale
Personal safety score	1661000286101	Personal safety score	Observable entity
Safe at home	1671000286105	I feel safe at home	Observable entity
Respected at home	1681000286107	I feel respected at home	Observable entity
Safe outside	1691000286109	I feel safe outside home	Observable entity
Respected outside	1701000286109	I feel respected outside home	Observable entity
Loneliness	1711000286106	Loneliness panel (How often do you)	Assessment scale
Loneliness score	1721000286103	Loneliness score	Observable entity
No one to talk to	1731000286101	Have no one to talk to?	Observable entity
Feel left out	1741000286107	Feel left out?	Observable entity
Feel alone	1751000286105	Feel alone?	Observable entity
Feel lonely	1761000286108	Feel lonely?	Observable entity
Patient experience	1791000286100	howRwe panel (How are we doing? – our recent care)	Assessment scale
howRwe score	1801000286101	howRwe score	Observable entity
Kindness	1811000286104	Treat you kindly	Observable entity
Listen/explain	1821000286107	Listen and explain	Observable entity
Prompt	1831000286109	See you promptly	Observable entity
Organised	1841000286103	Well organised	Observable entity
Service integration	1851000286100	Service integration panel (How well do services work together)	Assessment scale
Integration score	1861000286102	Service integration total score	Observable entity
Services talk together	1871000286106	Services talk to each other	Observable entity
Service knowledge	1881000286108	Staff know what other services do	Observable entity

(continued)

Table A3 (continued)

Name	SCT ConceptId	Preferred synonym	Hierarchy
Repeat story	1891000286105	I don't have to repeat my story	Observable entity
Services work together	1901000286106	Different services work well together	Observable entity
Privacy	1921000286100	Privacy panel (Thinking about how we use your data)	Assessment scale
Privacy score	1931000286103	Privacy score	Observable entity
Data is safe	1941000286109	My data is kept safe and secure	Observable entity
Data shared as needed	1951000286107	My data is only shared as needed	Observable entity
Can see/check data	1961000286105	I can see and check my data	Observable entity
Happy about data use	1971000286101	I am happy about how my data is used	Observable entity
Digital confidence	1991000286102	Digital confidence panel (Digital devices include computers smartphones & tablets)	Assessment scale
Digital confidence score	2001000286104	Digital confidence score	Observable entity
Digital usage	2011000286102	I use a digital device frequently	Observable entity
Peer usage	2021000286105	Most of my friends use digital devices	Observable entity
Access to help	2031000286107	I can usually get help if I am stuck	Observable entity
Confident digitally	2041000286101	I feel confident using most digital devices	Observable entity
Product confidence	2051000286103	Product confidence panel (How do you feel about [this product]?)	Assessment scale
Product confidence score	2061000286100	Product confidence score	Observable entity
Frequent user	2071000286109	I use it frequently	Observable entity
Confident user	2081000286106	I feel confident using it	Observable entity
Know benefits	2091000286108	I know the potential benefits	Observable entity
Know problems	2101000286103	I know potential problems	Observable entity
User satisfaction	2111000286101	User satisfaction panel (What do you think of [this product]?)	Assessment scale

(continued)

Table A3 (continued)

Name	SCT ConceptId	Preferred synonym	Hierarchy
User satisfaction	2121000286109	User satisfaction score	Observable entity
Helps me	2131000286106	It helps me do what I want	Observable entity
Easy to use	2141000286100	It is easy to use	Observable entity
Can get help	2151000286102	I can get help if I need it	Observable entity
Product satisfaction	2161000286104	I am satisfied with this product	Observable entity
Training	2171000286108	Training panel (Thinking about this course)	Assessment scale
Training score	2181000286105	Training score	Observable entity
Reaction	2191000286107	It was relevant and I enjoyed it	Observable entity
Learning	2201000286109	I have learnt new things	Observable entity
Behaviour	2211000286106	I shall use what I have learnt	Observable entity
Results	2221000286103	It will have a positive Impact	Observable entity

Index

A
Analysis, 13, 24, 26, 40, 55, 56, 59, 61, 63–65, 79, 81, 87, 114, 121, 122, 128, 131, 133, 134
Analysis, data of PROMs and PREMs, 56
Apgar, 13–15
Apgar score, 14
Application Program Interfaces (APIs), 67, 68, 71, 73, 79
Assessed need, 194, 197

B
Behavior change, 38, 39, 177, 184, 209, 214
  behaviour change, 39
  capability, 39
  opportunity, 39
  motivation, 39
Behavioral Change Techniques (BCTs), 38, 39
Bias, 42–47, 87, 114, 201
Bias, types of, 44
  cognitive bias, 45
  contextual bias, 45
  statistical bias, 45

C
Campaign to End Loneliness, 168, 175
Career progression, 55
Caregivers, 7, 39, 52, 102, 201–204
  case study, 202
Care home residents, 201, 204
Care provided, 101, 105, 108, 194, 197, 204
Carer, 6, 7, 102, 156, 161, 178, 194, 201
Case study, 60
  distribution, 116
    internal structure, 116
  impact, 117
    before and after, 118
    other measures, 118
Ceiling effect, 9, 23, 102, 116, 131

Change
  time period, 57
  individuals, 57
Change management, 31, 37, 38, 42, 186
CHEERS check-list, 63
Clinical interoperability, 67, 68
Coding Schemes, 80
  LOINC, 80
  SNOMED CT, 81
    computer-based, 82
    concepts, 81
    descriptions, 82
    reference terminology, 82
    relationships, 82
    value sets, 82
Codman, Ernest A., 13
Cognitive bias, 45
ColaborRATE, 149
COM-B, 38, 104, 153, 178, 184, 186, 196
Comment, 24, 113, 121, 122
Communication, 7, 33, 36, 58, 69–71, 105, 113, 118, 125, 180
Community, 6–9, 38, 64, 65, 73, 79, 85, 99, 101, 104, 107, 149, 166, 184
Compassion, 105, 113, 118
Complexity theory, 48
Computerized Adaptive Testing (CAT), 79, 80
Condition-specific measures, 8, 99, 139, 159, 160, 163
Consensus, 3, 16, 17, 46, 67–69, 88
Construct validation, 62, 173
Contact rate, 31, 32
Contextual bias, 45
Control, 6, 9, 41, 73, 108, 114, 145, 147, 150, 152, 165–167, 215
Cooperation rate, 31, 32
Core outcome sets, 99
Correlation, 62, 117–119, 132, 133, 137, 138, 143, 155, 172, 173

Index

Criteria, 8, 38, 41, 62, 72, 133, 136, 146, 153, 169, 170, 179, 186
Cronbach's α, 117, 132, 144, 154

D

Dashboard, 55, 56, 58, 60, 65
   dashboards for managers, 58
      before and after, 59
      demographics, 59
      downloads, 59
      periods, 59
      scores, 58
      thresholds, 59
Death rates, 85
Deaths of despair, 4, 85
De Jong Gierveld, 175
Demographics, 21, 22, 32, 36, 59, 63, 79, 122, 154, 161
Descriptive framework, 21, 22, 28, 121, 139
   comment, 24
   demographics, 21
   human role, 22
   item, 22
   measure, 22
   option, 23
   questionnaire, 21
   readability, 24
   readability measures, 24
   translations, 25
Development, 112
   devising Items, 112
      options, 113
      refining the items
      scope, 112
      sourcing items, 112
   readability, 115
   scoring, 114
Devising items, 112
Diagnosis Related Groups (DRGs), 5
Digital competence, 178, 179, 182, 187–189, 196, 199
Digital confidence, 105, 109, 177, 178, 181, 182, 189, 196, 217
Digital exclusion, 34
Dimension, 9, 14, 16, 22, 37, 46, 80, 81, 86, 113, 125, 128, 153, 165, 174, 178, 185, 196
Distribution, 9, 23, 27, 35, 59, 116, 117, 122, 126, 131, 132, 154, 179
Domain, 22, 42, 67, 74, 100, 101, 141, 160, 165, 166, 174, 178, 193

E

Early pioneers, 13
Education, 37, 45, 55, 85, 104, 107, 111, 113, 149, 154, 155, 165–167, 185, 210, 215
Effect size, 126, 134
EQ-5D, 18, 125, 127–129, 137–139
EQ-5D-3L, 125, 128, 129, 134, 136, 138
EQ-5D-5L, 92, 125, 129, 138
EQ health and wellbeing, 144
EQ-VAS, 125, 128, 129, 134, 136–138
EuroQoL, 125, 127
Exploratory factor analysis, 117, 144, 155, 173

F

FHIR manifesto, 71
FHIR resources, 73
Flesch-Kincaid grade, 24, 25, 33, 115, 138, 146, 147, 155, 163, 174, 175, 189, 190
Floor effect, 9, 23, 102, 116, 131
Friends and family test, 111, 118, 119, 121

G

General practice, 31, 32, 112, 177, 188, 189
General practice patient survey, 32, 111
Generic measures, 8, 9, 99, 112, 125–127, 139, 141, 153, 159, 167

H

Health confidence, 60, 101, 103, 107, 143, 149, 150, 152–155, 160, 163, 165, 169, 171–174, 194, 195, 202, 203, 209, 213
Health Confidence Score (HCS), 103, 143, 149, 151, 153–155, 172–174, 194, 209, 213
Health Index for England, 165, 166
Health inequalities, 45, 165
Health-related quality of life, 18, 103, 125
Health status, 4, 15–18, 60, 62, 63, 80, 87, 101–103, 106, 118, 119, 125–127, 129–131, 138, 139, 142–144, 150, 154, 155, 160, 162, 165, 169, 171–174, 194, 196, 201–204, 208, 212
   case study1, 131
      distribution of scores, 131
      internal structure, 132
      method, 131
      validity, 133
   EQ-5D, 127
   SF-36 and SF-12, 126

case study2, 133
    comparisons, 138
    correlations, 137
    results, 134
Health status measure – howRu, 129
History, 7, 11, 49, 72, 76, 162
HL7 FHIR, 67, 68, 70
Hospital Consumer Assessment of Healthcare Providers and Systems (HCAHPS), 111
Housing, 104, 108, 165–167, 174, 210, 215
HowRu, 80, 81, 102, 103, 118, 119, 125, 129–133, 138, 139, 143, 144, 153–155, 162, 172–174, 194, 202, 204, 208, 212

I

Impact evaluation, 153, 177
Incremental Cost-Effectiveness Ratio (ICER), 18, 133, 134
Individual care, 99, 101, 103, 107, 153, 194, 197
Individualised measures, 3, 8, 159, 160, 163
    comparisons of measures, 163
    MYCaW, 160
    person-specific outcome, 161
Individuals, 3, 5–7, 10, 19, 21, 22, 26, 35, 36, 38, 43, 46, 52, 55, 57, 64, 74, 76, 79, 86, 87, 89, 90, 93, 94, 101, 105, 111, 114–117, 118, 125, 132, 139, 144, 151, 154, 159, 160, 162, 165–167, 179, 180, 184, 194, 204, 207
Innovation, 8, 31, 34–38, 42, 43, 49, 52, 53, 99, 101, 105, 106, 109, 147, 177–180, 183–185, 187, 189, 190, 196, 198
Innovation-decision process, 36, 37, 180
Innovation evolution, 177
    case study—digital readiness in general practice, 188
    comparison of measures, 189
    measures, 178
        behaviour change, 184
        digital competence, 187
        digital confidence, 181
        innovation readiness, 179
        innovation process, 182
        product confidence, 187
        product satisfaction, 183
        training, 185
Innovation process, 177, 180, 182, 183, 189, 196, 199

Innovation readiness, 34, 177–179, 181, 189, 196, 198
Innovativeness, 34–36, 106, 179
Innovativeness spectrum, 31, 35, 178, 180, 196
    innovators, 35
    early adopters, 35
    early majority, 35
    late majority, 36
    laggards, 36
Inter-item correlations, 144, 154, 172
International Society for Pharmaco-economics and Outcomes Research (ISPOR), 18, 63
International Society for Quality of Life Research (ISOQOL), 18
Interoperability, 17, 51, 67–72, 80–82, 188, 207
    clinical interoperability, 68
    process interoperability, 68
    semantic Interoperability, 67
    technical interoperability, 67
    layers of, 68
        data layer, 68
        human layer, 68
        institutional layer, 68
        technology layer, 68
Interoperability economics, 69
Interoperability standards, 68
IPROMs, 159
Item, 5, 9, 21–28, 58, 60–63, 74–77, 79–81, 86, 99, 100, 102, 112–120, 125–128, 130–133, 138, 144–147, 151, 152, 154, 155, 157, 163, 166–175, 179, 181–185, 187, 189, 190, 193, 202, 203, 208–211

J

Job confidence, 194, 197, 204
Job roles, 56
    analysts, 56
    clinicians, 57
    managers, 56

K

Kirkpatrick model, 185

L

Layers of interoperability, 68
Length and readability, 174
Level noise, 44
Life expectancy, 17, 85, 87, 88, 91, 93, 95, 165
LOINC Codes, 207
LOINC Answers, 207

Load, 79, 85, 89, 90, 92–95, 130
Load model, 89
Logical Observation Identifiers Names and Codes (LOINC), 67, 68, 71, 80, 81, 207, 208–211
Loneliness, 101, 104, 108, 165, 168–172, 174, 175, 216
Loneliness and social contact, 168
   loneliness, 170
   loneliness measures, 168
   social contact, 169

M

Measure, 3, 5–10, 13–16, 18, 19, 21–26, 28, 31, 40, 43, 44, 49–51, 53, 57–62, 64, 79, 80, 85, 86, 94, 99–106, 111–117, 119, 120, 122, 125–127, 129–134, 136, 138, 139, 141–147, 149–157, 159, 161–163, 165–175, 177–179, 181, 183–190, 193–196, 201–204, 207, 210, 214
Measure Yourself Concerns and Wellbeing (MYCaW), 159–161, 163
Measure Yourself Medical Outcome Profile (MYMOP), 160, 161
Mental health, 144
   comparisons, 146
   ReQoL, 145
   WEMWBS, 145
Morbidity, 17, 85, 87–89, 93–95
Mortality rate, 14, 85, 89, 90, 165, 166, 168
My Health Confidence (MHC), 149, 151, 152, 154, 155

N

NASSS, 53
NASSS Framework, 43, 49, 50, 177
NASSS Framework, levels of, 49
   adopter, 52
   condition, 49
   embedding and adaption over time, 52
   organizations, 52
   technology, 51
   value proposition, 51
   wider context, 52
National Institute for Health and Clinical Excellence (NICE), 18, 87, 129
NHS PROMs programme, 134, 137
Nightingale, 13
Noise, 23, 24, 27, 42–44, 46, 47, 57, 87, 201
Noise, Types of
   level noise, 44
   occasion noise, 44
   stable pattern noise, 41
Normalisation Process Theory (NPT), 178, 182

O

Occasion noise, 44
Office of National Statistics (ONS), 104, 142–144, 165, 168, 170
ONS4, 103, 141–144, 147, 170, 202
Option, 6, 9, 21–25, 27, 43, 44, 46, 57, 70, 75, 81, 86, 91, 92, 100, 102, 106, 113–115, 120, 121, 125, 128, 131, 135, 138, 143, 145–147, 152, 155, 162, 163, 167–170, 174, 175, 179, 189, 190, 196, 202
Option set, 23, 28, 99, 101, 102, 193, 207
Outcome, 3–7, 9, 10, 13, 16–18, 37, 39, 40, 48–50, 52, 57, 63, 64, 72, 86, 88, 90, 91, 94, 99, 101–104, 106, 125, 126, 134, 144, 145, 149, 151, 155, 157, 160–163, 165–167, 169, 171, 175, 177, 178, 186, 190, 194, 197, 210, 214
Oxford Hip Score, 134, 135, 137, 139
Oxford Knee Score, 134, 137, 139

P

Patient activation, 150, 151
Patient Activation Measure (PAM), 59, 149, 151, 152, 155
Patient-centred care, 125, 163
   case study, 154
   CollaboRATE, 157
   comparison of measures, 155
   Health Confidence Score (HCS), 153, 154
      See also knowledge, self-management, access, shared decision-making
   measures, 151
      my health confidence, 152
      Patient Activation Measure (PAM), 151
   self-efficacy, 149
   shared decision-making, 155
   shared decisions, 157
   supported self-management, 149
Patient experience, 19, 60, 61, 105, 108, 111–120, 143, 165, 171–174
Patient Generated Index (PGI), 160
Patient-reported experience measures, 7, 111, 162
Patient-Reported Outcome Measures (PROMs), 3, 7, 8, 10, 11, 13, 15, 17–19, 21, 27, 28, 31, 35–39, 41–44, 50–53, 55–57, 61, 65, 67,

Index

72, 73, 99, 100, 101, 111, 114, 133, 134, 141, 153, 159, 160, 162, 163, 167, 169, 174, 177–179, 201, 207
  before 1980, 15
  1980s, 15
  1990s, 18
  2000s, 18
  academic societies, 18
  patient-reported outcomes, 17
  pharmaco-economics, 18
  QALYs, 17
Patient-reported outcomes, 17, 18, 99, 159, 167, 193
Patient safety, 19, 195, 198
PDSA cycle, 39, 40
  plan, 40
  do, 40
  study, 40
  act, 40
Personalised Care, 5
  person-centred care, 6
Personal Wellbeing Score (PWS), 41, 103, 141, 143–145, 147, 153, 163, 167, 172–174, 194, 202, 208, 212
Person-centred care, 6, 7, 150
Person-Reported Experience Measure (PREM), 3, 7, 8, 10, 11, 15, 18, 19, 21, 27, 28, 31, 35–39, 41–44, 51–53, 55–57, 61, 65, 67, 72, 73, 99, 100, 101, 111, 114, 141, 153, 159, 160, 163, 167, 177–179, 195, 201, 207
Person-Specific Outcome (PSO), 159, 161–163
Pharmaco-economics, 18
Poverty, 104, 108, 165–167, 174
Preference, 3, 11, 18, 26, 27, 46, 85–87, 89–91, 126, 129, 139, 207
Preference measures, 86
Privacy, 7, 22, 105, 108, 113, 195, 198, 217
Process, 4, 5, 8, 15, 21, 25, 26, 36–38, 51, 61, 62, 67–69, 72, 78, 87, 101, 111, 150, 151, 155, 157, 177, 178, 180, 182, 186, 189, 193, 196
Process interoperability, 68
Product confidence, 105, 109, 177, 178, 187–189, 196, 199, 217
Production of Care Systems, 5
Profile, 16, 67, 71, 73, 128
PROMs and PREMs, 7
  condition-specific measures, 8
  criteria applied to, 8
    brevity, 8
    clarity, 8
    generic, 9
    multi-attribute, 9
    multi-modal, 9
    psychometric properties, 9
    relevance, 9
    responsiveness, 9
Provider culture, 99, 101, 105, 108, 195, 198
Proxies, 22, 39, 76, 195, 201, 202
Publication check-list, 63

Q

QALY Model, 87
Quality Adjusted Life-Years (QALY), 13, 17, 18, 85, 87, 88, 90, 92–95, 125, 126, 128, 129, 133, 134
Quality Chasm, 4
Quality measures, 4
  types of information, 4
    structure, process, outcome, 4
Quality of life, 18, 46, 87–89, 99, 101, 103, 106, 125, 149, 151, 162, 194, 196, 201
Questionnaire, 7, 9, 21–24, 44, 67, 72–80, 112–114, 119, 121, 126, 134, 159, 160, 183, 202
  content, 74
  response, 74
Questionnaire resource, 67, 73–77, 79

R

Readability, 8, 21, 24, 25, 71, 115, 138, 146, 155, 163, 169, 174, 189
Recovering Quality of Life (ReQoL), 141, 144, 145, 147
Reducing noise and bias, 46
Refining the items, 112, 113
Relationships with other resources, 77
Reliability, 14, 35, 111, 113, 117
Representational State Transfer (REST), 71
Resource, 4–6, 15, 17, 41, 52, 64, 70–79, 142, 151, 159, 185
Response rate, 9, 10, 31–33, 39, 121, 122, 131, 193
RESTful APIs, 71
Role, 6, 22, 55–57, 65, 68, 72, 77, 78, 100, 104, 113, 126, 149, 151, 152, 156, 193, 194–195, 201
Rosser, R., 16, 95, 129

S

Scale, 5, 15, 16, 23, 26–28, 40, 41, 43, 44, 46, 47, 49, 58, 60, 81, 87–89, 94, 102, 114–116, 121, 125, 126, 128, 129, 131, 132, 134, 137, 139, 141,

143–146, 151, 152, 154, 157, 161, 162, 165, 167–169, 175, 177, 179, 181, 183, 184, 203, 204, 212–218
  interval, 28
  nominal, 28
  ordinal, 28
  ratio, 28
Schedule for Evaluation of Individual Quality Of Life (SEIQOL), 160
Scope, 55, 61, 80, 99, 111, 112, 114, 163, 183
Score, 14, 15, 24–27, 41, 43, 44, 47, 58–63, 73, 79–81, 86, 87, 102, 103, 114–122, 125, 126, 128, 131–134, 136–139, 143–147, 150–152, 154, 155, 161–163, 165–167, 169–175, 179, 182, 189, 190, 194, 202, 203, 208–218
Scoring, 14, 25, 62, 81, 114, 126, 129, 139, 144, 170, 179
Scoring scheme, 14, 21, 25, 28, 134, 139, 144, 153
  logarithmic scales, 27
  normative scales, 27
  preference weights, 27
  raw scores, 26
  thresholds, 27
  transformed scores, 27
  weight, 26
Self-efficacy, 108, 149–151, 154, 166, 167, 181, 182, 187
Semantic interoperability, 67, 80
Service integration, 105, 108, 111, 119, 120, 195, 197, 211, 216
Service provided, 99, 101, 105, 194, 197
SF-12, 27, 59, 125–127, 131, 133, 138, 139
SF-36, 18, 27, 59, 125–127, 138, 139
Shared Decision-Making (SDM), 6, 11, 101, 103, 113, 149, 153–157, 195, 209, 213
Shared decisions, 101, 104, 107, 149, 157, 195, 197, 198, 209, 213
Short Warwick-Edinburgh Mental Well-Being Scale (SWEMWBS), 141, 143, 145–147
SMART criteria, 41
  assignable, 41
  measurable, 41
  specific, 41
  realistic, 41
  time-bound, 41
SMART objectives, 41, 112
SNOMED CT, 51, 67, 68, 71, 80–82, 207, 212
SNOMED CT Codes, 207

Social contact, 104, 108, 165, 168–175, 210, 215
Social contact – case study, 171
Social determinants of health, 5, 101, 104, 165, 167, 171, 174, 210, 215
  Health Index for England, 165
  social determinants measure, 166
Social prescribing, 7, 60, 159–161, 163, 165–167, 169, 171–174
Sourcing items, 112
Spread, 28, 31, 34–36, 43, 49, 177, 178, 180, 185, 187
Stable pattern noise, 23, 44
Staff relationships, 195, 198
Staff-reported measures, 100, 101, 193, 194
  care provided, 194
    patient confidence, 195
    service integration, 195
    service provided, 194
  individual care, 194
    assessed need, 194
    job confidence, 194
  innovation, 196
    behaviour Change, 196
    digital competence, 196
    innovation process, 196
    innovation readiness, 196
    product confidence, 196
    user satisfaction, 196
    training, 196
  provider culture, 195
    patient safety, 195
    privacy, 195
    shared decisions, 195
    staff relationships, 195
    staff safety, 195
  quality of life, 194
    health status, 194
    person-specific outcome, 194
    work wellbeing, 194
Staff safety, 195, 198
Standard, 14, 18, 24, 27, 35, 36, 43, 44, 51, 59, 61, 63, 67–71, 111, 116, 117, 121, 126, 131, 134, 139, 143, 154, 155, 168, 170, 190
Standard gamble, 16, 86, 91, 92
Statistical bias, 45
Statistical packages, 61
Statistical packages validity, 61
Structure, 4, 5, 38, 46, 55, 56, 62, 73, 74, 81, 100, 101, 116, 117, 120, 126, 127, 132, 183, 193
Structured data, 72

Structured Data Capture, 73
Subjective wellbeing, 141, 142
    ONS4, 114
    PWS, 143
Supported self-management, 7, 149, 150
Survey, 10, 21, 24, 25, 31–33, 39, 43–47, 49, 51, 59, 72, 78–81, 95, 102, 106–109, 111, 115, 116, 122, 125, 126, 128, 131, 133, 141–143, 154, 163, 168, 171, 177, 178, 188, 190, 193, 196, 201, 202, 204

T
Taxonomy, 99, 100
    care provided, 105
        patient experience, 105
        service integration, 105
    individual care, 103
        acceptance of loss, 104
        adherence, 104
        behaviour change, 104
        community, 104
        health Confidence, 103
        loneliness, 104
        neighbour relationships, 104
        personal safety, 105
        self-Care, 103
        shared decisions, 104
        social contact, 104
        social determinants, 104
    innovation, 105
        digital confidence, 105
        digital readiness, 106
        product confidence, 105
        user Satisfaction, 106
        training, 106
    patient and staff-reported measures, 100
    option sets, 101
    PREMs Domains, 101
    PROMs Domains, 101
    provider culture, 105
        privacy, 105
    quality of life, 103
        fatigue, 103
        health status, 103
        personal wellbeing, 103
        person-specific outcome, 103
        sleep, 103
    table, 102

Technical interoperability, 67
Terminology binding, 67, 71
Threshold, 22, 27, 59, 63, 136
Timeliness, 113
Time periods, 55, 57, 59
Time trade-off, 16, 86, 91
Torrance, G., 16
Training, 16, 37, 55, 68, 106, 109, 113, 130, 159, 177, 178, 185, 186, 189, 196, 199, 218
Triple Aim, 6, 18, 19
Types of validity, 62

U
UCLA loneliness, 168
Use cases, 72
    data update, 72
    notification, 72
User satisfaction, 106, 109, 177, 178, 184, 189, 196, 199, 217, 218

V
Validity, 61
Value of a Statistical Life (VSL), 85–89, 142

W
Ware, 51
Warwick-Edinburgh Mental Well-Being Scale (WEMWBS), 145–147
Webhook, 71, 72
Weight, 26, 27, 46, 71, 87, 90, 93, 103, 107, 128, 129, 209, 213
Wellbeing, 6, 7, 41, 60, 61, 101, 103, 104, 106, 125, 141–143, 145–147, 160, 161, 165, 168, 171–174, 194, 202
Williams, A., 16, 95
Worked example, 90
    load for a hypothetical life, 94
    derivation of qaly, 92
    derivation of load, 92
    preference estimation, 90
    QALYs for a hypothetical life, 93
    surgery outcomes, 94
Workflow, 38, 77–80
    computerized adaptive testing, 79
    static forms, 79
Work wellbeing, 194, 196, 199

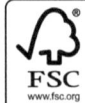

MIX
Papier aus verantwortungsvollen Quellen
Paper from responsible sources
FSC® C105338

If you have any concerns about our products,
you can contact us on
ProductSafety@springernature.com

In case Publisher is established outside the EU,
the EU authorized representative is:
**Springer Nature Customer Service Center GmbH
Europaplatz 3, 69115 Heidelberg, Germany**

Printed by Libri Plureos GmbH
in Hamburg, Germany